# FROM BIRTH TO FIVE YEARS

*From Birth to Five Years: Practical developmental examination* is a step-by-step 'how to' guide to the developmental examination of pre-school children. This book has been developed alongside the original *From Birth to Five Years: Children's developmental progress* as a companion volume that expands on the normative developmental stages outlined in Mary Sheridan's pioneering work in the field, by offering practical guidance for health, education and social care professionals, or anyone concerned with monitoring children's developmental progress.

This book is based on up-to-date research into current child development philosophies and practices, and aims to support the wider group of professionals who are required to assess children's developmental progress as part of their day-to-day working practices. The book begins with a practical framework for developmental examination, then progresses through each of the key developmental domains, offering guidance on enquiry and observation, and on how to chart typical and atypical patterns, with 'red flags' for recognising significant delay or disordered development. Advice is also given on how to make sense of the findings and how best to communicate this information to parents.

To consolidate and expand on the practical and theoretical information across this book and the original *From Birth to Five Years*, a new companion website is available at **www.routledge.com/cw/sharma**, which includes the following additional learning material:

- a timeline of the key developmental domains;
- introductions to theories of development, with links to further reading;

- further detail on topics signposted in the text;
- video clips demonstrating practical assessment skills.

**Ajay Sharma** is a Consultant Community Paediatrician at Guy's and St Thomas' NHS Foundation Trust, Southwark, London.

**Helen Cockerill** is a Consultant Speech and Language Therapist at the Evelina London Children's Hospital, Guy's and St Thomas' NHS Foundation Trust.

# FROM BIRTH TO FIVE YEARS

## Practical developmental examination

Ajay Sharma and Helen Cockerill

Illustrations by Nobuo Okawa

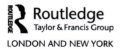

Routledge
Taylor & Francis Group

LONDON AND NEW YORK

First published 2014
by Routledge
2 Park Square, Milton Park, Abingdon, Oxon, OX14 4RN

and by Routledge
711 Third Avenue, New York, NY 10017

*Routledge is an imprint of the Taylor & Francis Group, an informa business*

*British Library Cataloguing in Publication Data*
A catalogue record for this book is available from the British Library

*Library of Congress Cataloging-in-Publication Data*
Sharma, Ajay, author.
  From birth to five years. Children's developmental progress /
  by Ajay Sharma and Helen Cockerill. — 4th edition.
    p. ; cm.
  Preceded by: From birth to five years: children's developmental progress /
  Mary D. Sheridan. 3rd ed. / rev. and updated by Ajay Sharma and
  Helen Cockerill. 2008.
  Complemented by: From birth to five years. Practical developmental
  examination / by Ajay Sharma and Helen Cockerill. 2014.
  Includes bibliographical references and index.
  I. Cockerill, Helen, author. II. Sheridan, Mary D. (Mary Dorothy).
  From birth to five years. 2008. Preceded by (work): III. Sharma, Ajay.
  From birth to five years. Practical developmental examination.
  Complemented by (work): IV. Title.
  [DNLM: 1. Child Development. 2. Child, Preschool. 3. Infant. WS 105]
  RJ131
  618.92—dc23                                        2013033534

ISBN13: 978-0-415-83458-2 (hbk)
ISBN13: 978-0-415-83459-9 (pbk)
ISBN13: 978-0-203-49181-2 (ebk)

Typeset in Univers by
Keystroke, Station Road, Codsall, Wolverhampton

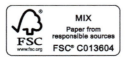
MIX
Paper from
responsible sources
FSC
www.fsc.org   FSC® C013604   Printed and bound by CPI Group (UK) Ltd, Croydon, CR0 4YY

# Contents

# A visual tour of the book

## Links to companion website

Whenever you see a boxed feature like this in the margin, with the @ symbol, look for the related supplementary material on the companion website ('Primitive and protective reflexes in infancy', in this example).

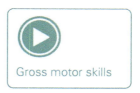

Whenever you see a boxed feature like this in the margin, with a 'play video' symbol, look for a related practical assessment skills instructional video on the companion website ('Gross motor skills', in this example).

## Further reading and references

Most chapters in the book conclude with a list of key scholarly books and articles, useful for practitioners to expand their knowledge of the theories and concepts covered, and helpful for students developing and researching essays and assignments. A full list of references is also included at the end of the book.

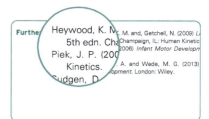

## Glossary

Key terms are highlighted in *italic* within the text, and defined in a comprehensive glossary at the end of the book.

# Introduction

When should we be concerned if parents or others think that a child is developing or behaving differently from other children? How do we know when the child needs help, and what kind of help should we give? These are the questions that face those working with children across a range of settings. There are many books that describe children's expected *developmental milestones*, but fewer resources on how to approach the assessment of an individual child's progress. This book provides a helpful guide for child health, education and social care practitioners who have responsibility for monitoring the development of children. It builds on the classic text, *Mary Sheridan's From Birth to Five Years: Children's developmental progress*, long recognised as an important source of information. This volume provides a structured approach to the examination of young children's abilities, rooted in current evidence-based understanding of the factors that influence development. It offers guidance on a stepwise process of enquiry, observation and making sense of findings.

**HOW TO USE THIS BOOK**

Practitioners working at different levels, from universal or primary care to targeted services for vulnerable children, can use the information and the method described here according to their level of competency and specific professional role to make sense of the child's needs, provide support and seek further assessment as required. For example, while some practitioners may only use the method to elicit concerns and explore the risk factors, others may use the method to make detailed enquiry and elicit developmental observations, and yet other practitioners may build on the information collated by undertaking a full physical examination and referral for investigations. *Red-flag* indicators described in Section 2 are useful pointers for seeking help.

Practical guidance (including video clips) for eliciting developmental observations, further information regarding some key concepts in child development, and references are all provided on the companion website. For most practitioners, learning about children's development is an ongoing process and further reading is recommended after each section.

# Conceptual framework

# A practical framework for developmental examination

Developmental examination is a part of the process of early identification of children's developmental difficulties. It is most meaningful when it builds on the developmental surveillance for all children and leads to further focused assessment, investigations, *facilitative guidance*, support and intervention (Table 1). Developmental examination is undertaken in response to parental

*Table 1* Process for identification of developmental needs.

|  | Objectives | Methods |
|---|---|---|
| **Surveillance: Universal: for all children** | Promoting health and development; promotion of good care and parenting; identification of risk factors; early presumptive identification of developmental difficulties. | Ongoing process involving parents (through the use of a personal child health record) and practitioners working with children at the universal level, e.g. child development workers, health visitors and general practitioners. |
| **Developmental examination** | To verify concerns, to elicit and categorise developmental function and any likely risk or impairment, provide support and guidance and arrange further assessment and/or investigations as required. | Clinical evaluation based on the knowledge of developmental progression and factors influencing it, skills and tools for eliciting concerns, history and making developmental observations. |
| **Developmental assessment: for established concerns** | To provide a detailed description of the child's developmental strengths and weaknesses for management planning and monitoring. | Standardised assessment methods used by paediatricians, psychologists and therapists, e.g. Griffith's or Bayley's scales. |
| **Diagnostic or functional assessment** | Diagnostic or functional assessment for management planning | Diagnostic tools, e.g. Autism Diagnostic Observations Schedule or functional assessment tools used by therapists. |

or other professionals' concerns regarding a child's function and/or behaviour and to proactively monitor progress in children with health or social risks.

The wide variation in ages at which typically developing children achieve *developmental milestones* may create difficulties in identifying children with vulnerabilities. Practitioners risk causing a delay in identification or falsely reassuring parents if they use subjective impressions to comment on the child's developmental progress (Glascoe and Dworkin 1993). Standardised tests of development differentiate children, comparing their performance to the expected *norms*, for their level of abilities or function. These tests are considered as gold standard by some but may be impractical in terms of time, unsuitable for the child's comprehension or motor abilities, and often too narrowly focused on *measuring* development (Greenspan and Meisels 1996).

Developmental examination may, on its own, lack the sensitivity and specificity of standardised assessments, but combined with the right knowledge, training and experience, and connected with the wider system of developmental surveillance, it has a useful place in promoting positive developmental outcomes. Developmental examination generally takes place when risks or concerns have been identified by parents or professionals. It enables professionals to identify any *vulnerability*, provide the required guidance and support, and access further detailed assessment and/or intervention services as required.

The structured developmental examination framework described here combines knowledge of the sequence of developmental progression* and an understanding of the processes influencing development (see Influences on development, p. 14 below), with the tools of systematic enquiry and observation. It provides a practical stepwise approach for eliciting concerns and *normative* and qualitative information about children's development. It provides a basis for identifying children who would benefit from support, by creating a focus on carers' concerns and the child's development, and guides practitioners in making further appropriate assessments and investigations.

*From Birth to Five Years – Children's Developmental Progress

The main components of this framework are:

A. Systematic enquiry of parents

   i.   eliciting concerns
   ii.  gathering information about the child's current abilities and function
   iii. identifying risks and protective factors

B. Observations

   i.   generic observations
   ii.  structured *domain-specific* observations/examination of developmental abilities, using age appropriate methods.

## A. SYSTEMATIC ENQUIRY

Gathering information from parents and carers is undoubtedly the most important aspect of evaluating development (Dooley *et al.* 2003). There are three main components of a systematic enquiry:

### i. Eliciting concerns

Parents, for various reasons, may not always bring up all their concerns (Box 1) (Glascoe and Marks 2011). A sensitive and supportive approach, starting first with open-ended questions and then following with more specific questions, is always helpful (see Communicating with parents/carers, p. 125). Well-elicited and carefully interpreted parental concerns guide practitioners in deciding the focus of further detailed enquiry, judging the need for parental assurance and advice and/or further examination or referrals. The sensitivity and specificity of systemically elicited concerns is as good (70–80 per cent) as standardised screening instruments for detecting developmental impairments (Glascoe 2003). Using a structured set of questions can elicit valid and useful responses (Table 2).

The significance of parental concerns changes with children's age. For example, concerns regarding general development, expressive language and social abilities are predictive of impairments at any age, while concerns regarding receptive language and motor function become more predictive of impairments after the age of 3 years (Tervo 2005). The relationship between parental concerns and the domain of impairment is not always direct: some concerns,

**BOX 1**  Barriers to parents raising concerns or accessing services

- Lack of awareness of children's developmental progress and/or of local services and how they can help

- Language barrier, social isolation

- Emotional and behavioural problems may be seen by some parents as moral, rather than psychological, deviations because of cultural beliefs (Katz and Pinkerton 2003)

- Parents living in poverty are more likely to be stressed and less likely to express concerns about their children (Elder *et al.* 1985)

- Stigma of a label or being seen as a 'failed parent'

- Lack of trust or suspicion

*Table 2*  Questions for eliciting concerns.

Do you have any concerns about how your child talks and makes speech sounds?

Do you have any concerns about how your child understands what you say?

Do you have any concerns about how your child uses his or her hands to do things?

Do you have any concerns about how your child walks or runs?

Do you have any concerns about how your child behaves?

Do you have any concerns about how your child gets along with others?

Do you have any concerns about how your child does things for him or herself?

Do you have any concerns about your child's learning?

Do you have any concerns about your child's hearing or vision?

Do you have any other concerns?

Source: Glascoe (1999).

such as poor language or social abilities, may also indicate *global developmental delay* or learning disability (Tervo 2005; Glascoe 1994). The onset and course of concerns, including any regression, should always be noted.

During the parental interview age-appropriate toys should be available for the child to explore. This will serve the purposes of helping the child to relax prior to examination of developmental abilities, allowing the practitioner to make some general observations, and distracting the child's attention from the carer's comments. However, some carers may have things they wish to say out of the child's hearing.

Parents are good at describing their pre-school child's current abilities and function, and their descriptions are sensitive indicators of the child's developmental status (Glascoe and Sandler 1995) Asking open-ended questions (Table 3) and then requesting examples elicits the most reliable history. Sample questions, specific to each domain of development, are given later in this volume.

**ii. Gathering information about the child's current abilities and function**

Information on relevant biological and family-social risk factors is gathered from parents and from the child's personal health record or other records/sources. Parents should be given reasons, and permission obtained, for gathering such information as some of it may be of a personal and sensitive nature. Children with multiple risk factors are at a higher risk for poor developmental outcomes, and support and guidance may need to focus on risk and protective factors rather than on any apparent developmental delay (see Promoting, protective and risk factors, p. 23).

**iii. Identifying risks and protective factors**

Practitioners working with children in any environment, in the natural setting of home or in a nursery/school or during a structured examination in a clinic, can make useful generic qualitative observations of children's behaviour and functional abilities. The usefulness of such observations improves if:

**B. OBSERVATION/ EXAMINATION**

**i. Generic observations**

a. these are recorded with some description of the context, e.g. where and when the behaviour was noted and, where appropriate, what preceded and followed a behaviour;

*Table 3* Generic enquiry of parents.

| Question | Focus of enquiry | Further investigation |
| --- | --- | --- |
| **What is your child like to live with?** | Whether the child is happy or unhappy, tearful or irritable, compliant or defiant, cooperative or oppositional, fearful/anxious/worried. Level of activity and impulsiveness. | Enquire about exactly what is the concern, its onset, duration, any particular situation that leads to the behaviour, parents' usual response to such behaviour and the consequences of a usual episode – what does the behaviour eventually lead to? |
| **Does your child sleep well?** | Poor sleep pattern can have a detrimental effect on the child's behaviour and can seriously affect parenting and family function. | A sleep diary should be used if there are any concerns regarding pre-sleep routine, time of falling asleep, number of times the child wakes up and for how long, what do the parents do, time the child gets up in the morning and any daytime naps. |
| **Is your child generally healthy?** | Current health status, any treatment and any behaviour suggestive of a seizure disorder such as periods of altered awareness, consciousness or abnormal movements. | Observation should be made of nutritional status including weight and height check, using appropriate growth charts. |
| **Any recent changes in the social or health circumstances of family members?** | Changes in a child's abilities and functioning may arise from instability in the home. | Liaison with general practitioner/other service providers (e.g. nursery, social services). |
| **Has your child ever lost any skills?** | Any change in current abilities, function or behaviour, e.g. speech, mobility, hand function, bowel/bladder function. | **Any loss of function, previously acquired, should lead to a full general and neurological assessment.** (see Plateauing or regression, p. 120) |
| **Do you think your child's abilities are broadly in line with other children of the same age?** | Pattern of development across all domains including independence, self-care abilities of eating, toileting, dressing/undressing. | May stimulate more detailed questions about specific areas of development when enquiring about domain-specific abilities. |

b. actions rather than intentions are recorded, e.g. 'the child repeatedly put the car in his mouth' rather than 'the child was seeking sensory stimulation';

c. assumptions are avoided, e.g. 'the child took the car from another child' rather than 'the child was not friendly with another child';

d. opinions are separated from observations, e.g. 'the child did not interact with other children' rather than 'the child was upset and did not want to play with other children'.

Some useful dimensions of generic behaviours (Figure 1) to observe are:

1. parent–child interaction: parents' awareness of the child's interests and actions, their interest in the child, response to the child's actions and negativity or praise (see Observing parent–child interaction, p. 72);

2. the child's *attention*: how well the child focuses on the activities, perseveres or completes any task and listens to the direction given (see Attention, impulsivity and activity level, p. 94);

3. general physical activity levels during the assessment;

4. any *impulsivity* – interrupting, snatching or randomly shifting from one activity to another;

5. child's mood (affect): happy/sad/flat/anxious – about any specific aspect or generally (see Emotional regulation and behaviour, p. 98);

6. the child's social awareness: how does the child relate to those present? Awareness, sharing, initiating interactions and responding to other's approaches (see Social behaviour and play, p. 85);

7. any change in the child's performance or behaviour with time or with the type of activities, e.g. on non-verbal tasks with toys during verbal interactions.

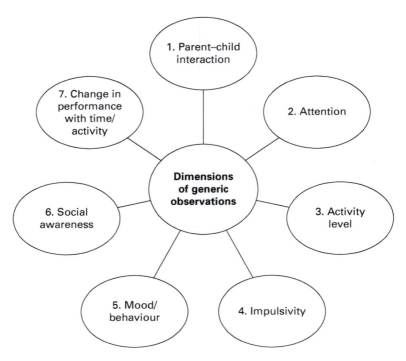

**Figure 1** *Dimensions of generic observations.*

**ii. Structured domain-specific observations/ examination**

During a structured examination developmental abilities are elicited, using age and domain-appropriate materials in a systematic manner, relating these findings to the knowledge of children's developmental progression. Such examination often takes place in clinical settings, but, given the appropriate materials, it can take place in any suitable uncluttered environment. Some guiding principles which underpin such observations are:

■ Awareness that both parents and children may be anxious and worried. Sufficient time should be given for the child to settle. It may be helpful to start with informal observations with the use of age-appropriate toys and other play material.

■ Simultaneous information is gathered about multiple domains of development even though the findings are described in specific domains of development for the purposes of structure and clarity of description. For example, any non-verbal task gives information about visual perception, fine and gross motor skills and cognitive skills; likewise responses on verbal tasks combine social, speech-language-communication and cognitive skills.

- Making note of qualitative information, i.e. how a task is done, is crucial rather than being over-focused on success/failure in a domain-specific activity. This should be made explicit to carers who may be anxious about the child's performance and regard the tasks as pass/fail tests.

- Motivation and transitions should be managed by structuring the setting to reduce distractions, doing one task at a time and praising the child's participation, not simply success in a given task.

- Any directions to the child should be appropriate to the developmental level, should be simple and active, e.g. 'look at the –' vs. 'show me –'. Verbal instructions can be with gestures where required to focus the child's attention, e.g. saying 'listen' with a gesture of listening with the ear, 'look' with the gesture of pointing from the eye to the relevant object.

A systematic approach to the structured examination for specific domains is described in Section 2. There is an unavoidable degree of overlap in the methods of enquiry between the domains, which is a reflection of the complexity and inter-relatedness of aspects of children's development.

Responding to concerns regarding a child's developmental progress requires:

**Pathway of care for children with developmental difficulties**

1. listening to parental concerns, making a detailed enquiry, conducting a developmental and physical examination and arranging investigations as indicated;

2. analysing or 'making sense' of the information at each step of the process. This means not simply describing the findings, but asking the question 'why' regarding any *vulnerability*;

3. working in collaboration with parents and other professionals to think and plan about what can be done to address the child's needs (care plan).

The following chapters in this book aim to provide the knowledge and information needed to take decisions and work through the suggested outline pathway (Figure 2).

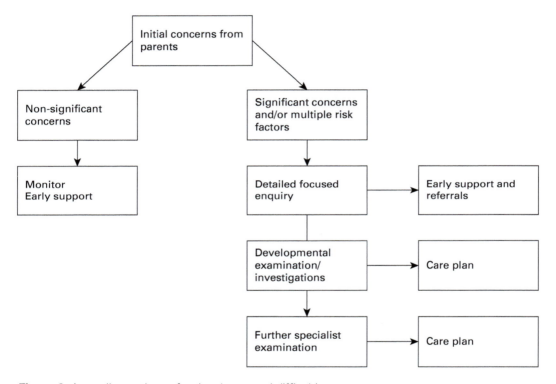

**Figure 2** *An outline pathway for developmental difficulties.*

Hobart, Christine, Frankel, Jill and Walker, Miranda (eds) (2009) *A Practical Guide to Child Observation and Assessment*, 4th edn. Cheltenham: Nelson Thornes.

A practical book with examples of observations and techniques, for professionals working in early years childcare.

Sheridan, Mary, Howard, Justine and Alderson, Dawn (2011) *Play in Early Childhood: From Birth to Six Years*. Abingdon: Routledge.

A classic introductory text to play and development – key topics for all those who work with young children. Updated for a contemporary audience and fully evidence-based, it explains how children's play develops and how they develop as they play.

Woolraich, M. L., Drotar, D. D., Dworkin, P. H. and Perrin, E. C. (2008) *Developmental Behavioural Pediatrics: Evidence and Practice*. Philadelphia, PA: Mosby Elsevier.

A textbook to help practitioners reach the right diagnostic and therapeutic decisions for children with developmental and psychological difficulties.

**Further reading**

# Influences on development

Development is a process of growth and transformation through which children achieve new physical, cognitive and psychological abilities. It enables them to become mobile, use their hands to do fine motor tasks, communicate, socialise, learn and become a productive member of society. Development creates both novelty – learning of new skills, and diversity – the wide range of variation seen in the rate and range of development.

The following questions arise in seeking to understand this process of change and growth: How does development progress? What moves development forward and causes the variation? How do nature (our genes) and nurture (our experience) work together to shape and drive development? Is development open to change through intervention?

## A DYNAMIC PROCESS OF CHANGE

During development change and growth happen simultaneously at multiple levels. These dimensions of change continually interact and pull each other forward:

■ *Genetic expression*: different genes 'come on line', 'switch on or off' or are expressed. This process is influenced by age and experience.

■ Brain growth: neural growth and connectivity are influenced by genes, age and experience.

■ Psychological processes: attention, memory, self-regulation – emotional and behavioural.

■ Knowledge and skills: perceptual, cognitive, linguistic and social.

■ Physical growth and ability.

Genes provide a template for the structure of brain and body. They are like sets of chemical instruction manuals that we pass from generation to generation through our chromosomes. Genes contain instructions for building proteins, enzymes and hormones. A gene works in concert with other genes – a single gene is rarely necessary or sufficient for a particular personal or developmental characteristic.

**GENES –
NATURE'S
TOOLS**

Genes affect development through:

a. direct effects on neural structure or connectivity;
b. increasing or decreasing production of *neurotransmitters*; and
c. increasing or decreasing susceptibility to the environment.

The action of a gene is not a fixed given. Whether a particular gene would be 'switched on or off' at a particular stage of development depends on environmental triggers – known as *epigenetic effects*. There is growing evidence that the epigenetic process is influenced by experience, diet and hormones (Hertzman 2011). It affects all children, not just those exposed to the extremes of abnormal environments (Rutter 2006). It enables the genetic template to come into being and then actively shapes it – creating both novelty and diversity (Figure 3).

What is the environment and how does it affect development? The 'environment' is made up of multiple levels – parents, family, neighbourhood and society, as well as the child's physical living space (Bronfenbrenner and Morris 2006). It is the 'crucible' for development where the essential ingredients of nurturing, protecting and experience interact with the genetic potential to forge the course of the developing child.

**Environmental
influences –
the movers and
shakers of
development**

Children's interactions with parents have an important role in shaping development. These interactions encourage, invite and engage a child and so provide nurturing experiences. The parent–child relationship depends on parents' temperament, experiences and resourcefulness, but it is also shaped by the child's own behaviour and the living environment of the family (Shonkoff and Phillips 2000). For example, psycho-social adversity, created by instability and chaos in the family or neighbourhood, can seriously jeopardise the parent–child relationship.

**Nurturing
environment –
positive
parent-child
interactions**

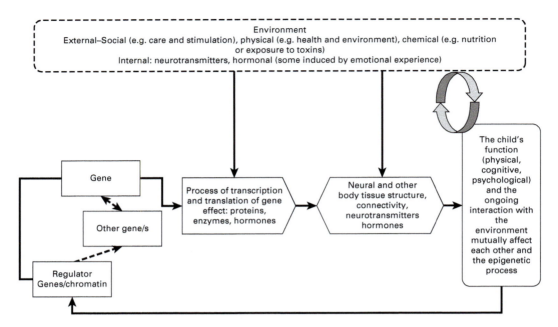

**Figure 3** *The genes, the environment and the child are all active agents for developmental progress.*

The 'sensitive-responsiveness' from parents is the most development-enhancing aspect of their interactions with the child. Generally, children who receive affectionate, *sensitive-responsive parenting* make better developmental progress, have better social skills and develop secure attachment with their parents (Glascoe and Leew 2010; Guralnick 2006).

**Learning environment – appropriately stimulating**

Exploration and play with developmentally appropriate toys and materials, spontaneous verbal interactions involving the child, and family routines such as social mealtimes and bedtime reading are important experiences which promote positive development. The relationship between the environmental effects and outcomes is non-linear, e.g. low levels of stimulation may not provide enough impetus for development and high levels of stress, e.g. created by overcrowding and high noise levels, may overwhelm the system (Lerner *et al.* 2011).

Adequate nourishment, prevention of illnesses (immunisation) and protection from violence or exposure to violence are the essential and basic needs of a developing child. Parental monitoring and support ensure safety and enhance peer relationships. Safe, healthy and happy children make better developmental progress.

Scientific studies are beginning to reveal the processes which make the environment 'get under the skin' and create lasting changes in brain structure and function. These changes affect children's psychological and emotional well-being and their developmental progress.

## HOW DOES THE ENVIRONMENT AFFECT DEVELOPMENT?

Neurons undergo proliferation and then migrate to different areas of the brain during gestation and the *perinatal period*. At this stage they are susceptible to injury from toxins, e.g. maternal alcoholism, radiation and infections such as rubella and HIV, which can cause learning disabilities and seizures.

**Effects on developing brain structure and function**

Neuronal connectivity or synapse formation, followed by some fine-tuning of the connectivity, takes place mostly during the first 2 years, though some areas such as the pre-frontal cortex (concerned with self-regulation) continue to mature till adolescence (Couperus and Nelson 2006). Early environmental experiences, such as visual stimulation and exposure to speech, are essential for the right connections to be made – as expressed in the well-known aphorism 'use it or lose it'. New synaptic connections or neuronal networks continue to be formed in response to unique individual experience, such as learning a musical instrument or exposure to multiple languages, and create inter-individual differences.

Early experience 'programmes' some biological responses, e.g. the Hypothalamic Pituitary Adrenal (HPA) axis regulates the secretion of hormones and steroids in response to stress, which in turn affects the formation of brain connectivity and responsiveness. Early persistent environmental stress such as neglect and abuse causes abnormally heightened HPA axis responsiveness and has 'toxic effects' on neuronal connectivity and function (National Scientific Council on the Developing Child 2005).

**Effects on regulatory abilities**

**Learning to regulate emotions**

Establishing selective and discriminating relationships with carers is also related to the capacity for emotional regulation, and the emergence of social competence (Sroufe 2005). Such experiences continue to affect children's attention, memory and other *executive functions*, located in the pre-frontal cortex, right up to adolescence.

**Effects on learning**

Environmental rewards positively reinforce the most adaptive behaviours (*operant conditioning*), creating a strong basis for learning from experience. With age children become less reliant on external rewards as their sense of satisfaction and self-pride become an *intrinsic reinforcement* for further learning. Learning also occurs on watching someone else behave in a certain way (modelling or observational learning). However, children do not just simply learn to copy others' behaviour: they interpret and learn the underlying pattern or rule and apply it to different situations to solve problems (Bandura 1989).

During certain periods some aspects of development are uniquely and optimally sensitive to specific types of experience or the effects of experience are particularly strong (*sensitive periods*), such as exposure to speech sounds for speech perception during the first year and binocular vision for intact visual perception during the pre-school years. Developmental change, in response to experience and engagement, however, happens at any age, though the intensity required for the experience to be effective may increase with age (Knudsen 2004).

**GENE-ENVIRONMENT INTERACTION**

Some children may be made more or less prone to express a genetic *vulnerability* depending on the environment being challenging or supportive. Many people may carry a trait for genetic vulnerability or strength but only some may develop a problem or strength depending on their experiences (Boyce and Ellis 2005). For example, people are genetically different in the level of enzyme monoamine oxidase (MAOA); those with low levels of the enzyme are at higher risk for aggressive and antisocial behaviour in adult life if they were abused as children as compared to those with high levels (Munafò *et al.* 2009).

Children's biological and psychological predisposition and the environment interact or transact with each other continuously and reciprocally to create new levels of learning, skills and resources – this is known as a *transactional process*. The 'changed' child then selects, perceives and interacts with the environment differently.

The environment changes in tandem with the child. Opportunities, expectations and challenges all vary over time, giving rise to new experiences, which further stimulate new developments in the child. The child and the environment are thus inextricably linked – they change and grow together as a dyad (Sameroff and Fiese 2000). The child is an active participant in this process through his/her choices and actions and becomes both the product and the producer of development.

Cultural variables such as shared values, expectations, beliefs and patterns of personal and social relationships, as expressed in daily routines, work together as a system influencing each other and the developing child in a *dynamic* manner. Cultural memory, traditions and practices show both continuity and change with time. Socio-economic factors and wider socio-political environments affect how people put their cultural values into practice. Children bring their own interpretations and responses, based on their ability and temperament, to successfully adapt to their environment, which for many children involves growing up with multiple sets of cultural values and practices. Children are not simply recipients of a culture; they actively influence and change the culture as well.

Super and Harkness (1997) describe three related components of the culturally influenced proximal environment:

1. the physical and social settings in which the child lives;

2. the culturally regulated child-rearing and socialisation practices; and

3. the psychological characteristics of the child's parents, especially their knowledge and beliefs about the process of child development and their emotional and social orientation to the tasks of child-rearing.

## THE CHILD AND THE ENVIRONMENT

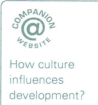

How culture influences development?

## CULTURAL INFLUENCES ON DEVELOPMENT

Interpretations of parent or child behaviour, based on the assumption of homogeneity of cultural practices within some ethnic or socio-economic groups, are likely to be misplaced as there are significant within-group differences in the cultural variables and how they are practised. It is often unproductive to focus on an individual cultural variable and its causal influence because multiple variables work together as a system; the impact of the same variable, e.g. a belief or a parenting style, depends on a wider set of social and cultural practices (Cole and Packer 2011).

There are wide-ranging influences of culture on language, social, cognitive and psychological development. Health and social care practitioners may lack awareness of the heterogeneity of cultural practices. There is a need to avoid incorrect assumptions, value judgements and the biases that may affect observations and interpretations of children's behaviour and learning (Rogoff 2003). Lack of knowledge in this area can create an environment of cultural mismatch between practitioners and families, reducing access and engagement for carers, and a risk of erroneous interpretation of the child's needs. A culturally sensitive system of care includes behaviours, attitudes and policies that enable practitioners to work effectively in cross-cultural situations. A framework for cultural competence has been described by Mason (1995).

## EMERGENCE OF NEW SKILLS IN DEVELOPMENT – THE SYSTEMS APPROACH

The systems approach (Thelen and Smith 2006) proposes that the emergence of novelty – new forms and function – occurs through interaction between different parts of the developing system and self-organisation of the emerging patterns. Every new and sustained perceptual and social experience triggers new brain connectivity and refines existing structure and behaviour. Even seemingly mundane skills are the foundations for later competencies: for example, early crawling experience leads to later wariness of heights and early verbal communication is linked to later understanding of others' mental states.

## PLASTICITY

There is a relative *plasticity* in development: the strength of influence of the environment at various points during the development of a skill depends on the timing, existing skills and the intensity and duration of new experiences. It is easier to learn some new competencies such as speaking a second language in early child-hood but, depending on the exposure and motivation, it can be learnt at any stage. Motivation, often spurred by the *social network* around the child, is of great help as most learning takes place in a social *context* (Rutter 2011).

There is a broad range of individual differences in development across all domains, which often makes it difficult to distinguish normal variations from transient or permanent impairments. Large inter-individual variation, often described as 'normative variation' and represented as a bell-shaped curve (Figure 4), is seen in all aspects of development – no two children, even in the same family, are similar.

## VARIATION IN DEVELOPMENT

A combination of genetic predisposition (minor genetic variations) and environmental adversity creates the variation in the 'typical' range, including the lower end of the normative graph, which includes children with lower levels of cognitive abilities, within the mild to moderate range. Children within this range of variation can change quite significantly in their abilities over time and there is

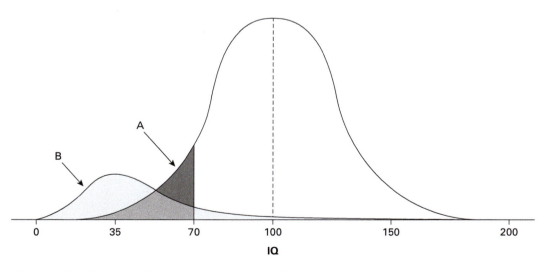

**Figure 4** *Distribution of (A) normative variation resulting in mainly mild-moderate degrees of cognitive impairment and (B) non-normative or pathological variation resulting in mainly severe and lasting cognitive impairment (based on Zeigler and Hodapp 1986).*

much movement between the 'typical' range and the 'mild' and 'moderate' impairment groups over time. This shift or movement reflects a child's developmental adaptation and is influenced by the risk and protective factors for that child (Sameroff 2009).

Severe and lasting impairments on the other hand are generally caused by organic disorders such as severe mutation of a single gene, *chromosomal disorders*, prenatal or postnatal infections and physical or toxic brain injury. Sometimes early, severe and persistent environmental deprivation can also cause severe and lasting impairment, with qualitative differences in the patterns of development.

Sometimes children show aetiology-specific patterns of behaviour, e.g. stereotypic hand wringing in Rett's syndrome, and specific patterns of development, e.g. strength in simultaneous processing of information as compared to a weakness in sequential processing in Fragile X and Prader-Willi syndromes. A wide range of variation in function is common, both within the group of children with severe impairment and within the different domains of development for an individual, depending on the type and degree of genetic, physical or environmental adversity and timing and intensity of environmental support.

**Further reading**

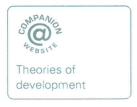

Theories of development

Cowie, H. (2012) *From Birth to Sixteen: Children's Health, Social, Emotional and Linguistic Development*. Abingdon: Routledge.
Keating, D. P. (ed.) (2012) *Nature and Nurture in Early Child Development*. Cambridge: Cambridge University Press.
McCartney, K. and Phillips, D. (eds) (2006) *Early Childhood Development*. Oxford: Blackwell Publishing.

# Promoting, protective and risk factors

Children develop to the best of their ability when they grow up in an environment which is safe, caring and nurturing and meets their individual needs, i.e., which is suitable for the child's ability, temperament and any specific health or learning needs (Shonkoff and Phillips 2000). The ongoing interactions between the child's intrinsic characteristics and the external environment create a spectrum from positive to negative outcomes and from resilience to *vulnerability* (Figure 5). This relationship is not direct or linear,

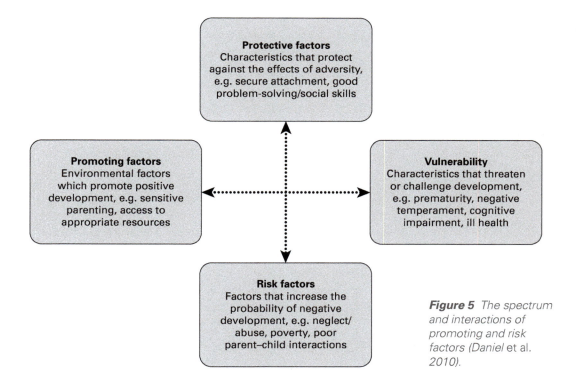

**Protective factors**
Characteristics that protect against the effects of adversity, e.g. secure attachment, good problem-solving/social skills

**Promoting factors**
Environmental factors which promote positive development, e.g. sensitive parenting, access to appropriate resources

**Vulnerability**
Characteristics that threaten or challenge development, e.g. prematurity, negative temperament, cognitive impairment, ill health

**Risk factors**
Factors that increase the probability of negative development, e.g. neglect/abuse, poverty, poor parent–child interactions

*Figure 5* The spectrum and interactions of promoting and risk factors (Daniel et al. 2010).

but probabilistic, i.e. positive or negative outcomes are not predicted, but their chances are relatively increased or decreased (Rutter 2011).

**PROMOTING AND PROTECTIVE FACTORS**

Promoting factors:

a. universal environmental resources or assets that generally promote positive development for all children (Masten and Gewirtz 2006), e.g. sensitive and responsive parenting, safe, stable and nurturing environment; or
b. environmental features that promote specific aspects of development, e.g. practice with fine motor tasks promotes fine motor skills.

Protective factors that mitigate the detrimental effects of risks are:

a. biological characteristics of a child, e.g. good memory, good problem-solving skills, outgoing temperament; or
b. characteristics of a child's environment which support better outcomes even in the face of adversity, such as alternative carers, supportive and resourceful family and a stable loving relationship (Bada *et al.* 2012).

Those working with children have a responsibility to proactively encourage promoting factors and, if there is adversity, support the protective factors in the environment.

**RISK FACTORS**

Risk factors increase the probability of poor psychological (cognitive and emotional) and social outcomes. Most of the poor developmental outcomes in children have their origin in early effects on the developing brain, particularly in the context of a paucity of promoting or protective factors (Shonkoff *et al.* 2012). Some risk factors are more strongly associated with particular outcomes, e.g. domestic violence with child maltreatment, early-onset conduct problems with later substance abuse and family history of criminal activity with youth offending; however, the risk factors overlap to a very large degree for most negative outcomes (Youth Justice Board for England and Wales 2005). The risk factors

*Table 4* Risk, promoting and protective factors.

|  | Risk factors | Promoting and protective factors |
| --- | --- | --- |
| **Child** | ■ Prenatal exposure to drugs, alcohol, infections<br>■ Prematurity, low birthweight<br>■ Neurological, sensory deficit<br>■ Poor nourishment, iron deficiency<br>■ Difficult temperament<br>■ Poor self-regulation<br>■ Delayed development | ■ Cognitive abilities<br>■ Social skills<br>■ Attachment with family/carer<br>■ Positive attitude and coping ability<br>■ Self-regulation |
| **Parents and family** | ■ Poor parenting, e.g. rejecting, neglecting, harsh or abusive<br>■ Lack of developmentally appropriate opportunities or space<br>■ Parental poor mental health/learning difficulties<br>■ Low maternal education<br>■ Parental/family conflict, domestic violence<br>■ Overcrowding at home | ■ Sensitive, warm and responsive parenting<br>■ Competent and stable carers<br>■ Breastfeeding<br>■ Adequate family resources and housing |
| **Social network** | ■ Lack of support for the family<br>■ Lack of peer group/isolation<br>■ Exposure to violence | ■ Supportive extended family/friend network<br>■ Regular participation in cultural or faith-based community activities<br>■ Access to playgroup, childcare, education, health services |
| **Community environment** | ■ Unemployment<br>■ Poor housing<br>■ Exposure to toxins, e.g. lead<br>■ Disadvantaged neighbourhood | ■ Provision of facilitative universal programmes, e.g. Sure Start, early education, family support |

Sources: Rutter (2013), Roulstone *et al.* (2011), Harrison and McLeod (2010), Martinez-Torteya *et al.* (2009) Evans (2006), Sameroff *et al.* (1993).

listed in Table 4 are generally associated with poor developmental, learning or behavioural outcomes during early childhood.

Most of the effects on a developing child are mediated by processes close to the child, such as parent–child interaction, childcare and stimulation. The common pathways effects on development (Figure 6) are through:

**How do these risks operate and why do have a long-lasting impact?**

a. insensitive parent–child interaction, e.g. coercive, intrusive or controlling interactions;

b. reduced learning opportunities, e.g. impoverished use of language for communication;

c. learning of negative behaviours, e.g. aggressive or antisocial behaviours;

d. genetic inheritance from parents, e.g. for some cognitive or psychological problems.

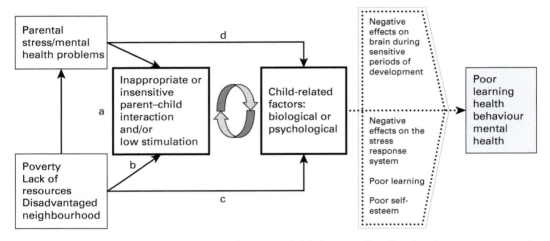

**Figure 6** *Interaction of biological and environmental risk factors affecting development.*

These effects become embedded or 'get under the skin' in the biological system of the child (National Scientific Council on the Developing Child 2005) by:

a. creating permanent or long-lasting effects during sensitive periods of development, e.g. effects of alcohol intake during pregnancy; attachment difficulties;

b. cumulative effects of recurrent neglect/abuse resulting in chronic activation of the stress response system, which causes ongoing damage to the structure and function of the brain (National Scientific Council on the Developing Child 2005);

c. affecting the outcome through a cascade effect, e.g. language problems in early childhood contributing to later emotional and behavioural difficulties, leading to harsh and restrictive parent-ing, which may in turn lead to truancy and youth offending (Lindsay and Dockrell, 2012);

d. chronic ill health resulting from poor nutrition or environmental toxins, e.g. lead.

While single or isolated negative environmental factors may have only a small, incremental effect, multiple risk factors make a major contribution to developmental problems (Figure 7) (Sameroff *et al.* 1993; Barth *et al.* 2007).

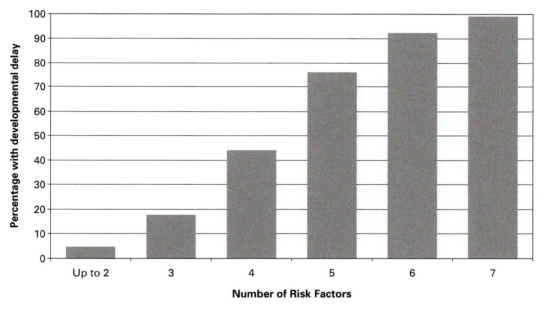

***Figure 7*** *Percentage of children with developmental delay by the number of risk factors present (Barth* et al. *2007).*

Early and persisting adversity – such as poverty, abuse or neglect, parental substance abuse or mental illness, and exposure to violence – can have a cumulative toll on an individual's physical and mental health (Figure 8) (Shonkoff *et al.* 2012). Risk factors com-monly co-occur, and when they do, poor outcomes, e.g. substance abuse, depression, heart disease and diabetes, are more likely (Martinez-Torteya *et al.* 2009).

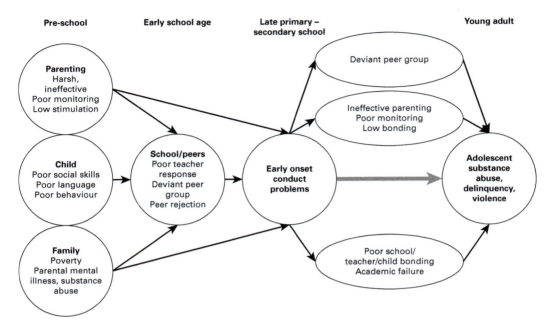

**Figure 8** *Compounding effects of multiple and persisting risk factors (Webster-Stratton and Taylor 2001).*

**Vulnerability**

While protective factors buffer against the risks, vulnerability factors accentuate their effects by making children more susceptible to adversity. These characteristics may be:

a. genetically based, e.g. children with disinhibited or fearful temperament may evoke or select situations which cause further damage to their development;

b. biologically based, e.g. *premature* children showing poorer outcomes in adverse conditions compared to children born at full term;

c. created by early experiences during periods of development when the adaptive systems are emerging, e.g. early persistent stresses in unsupported environments create altered reactivity of the stress response system, which becomes hyper-reactive to any stress in the future (Masten and Gewirtz 2006: 32);

d. related to their stage of development, e.g. children show fluctuating levels of vulnerability to social or physical adversity depending on their age: for example, in early infancy developing brains are more likely to be affected by social deprivation and iron deficiency; children also become more vulnerable to adverse experience during phases of transition, e.g. school entry and puberty.

Better understanding of risk, vulnerability, promoting and protective factors has provided an improved framework for prevention and intervention (Garner *et al.* 2012), by shifting focus from disease or deficit towards improving promoting factors and providing anticipatory guidance and interventions. Most situations require a combined approach of (a) taking a positive stance to promoting development and (b) maintaining an ongoing awareness of risks and vulnerabilities and taking timely actions for any concerns. Some general guiding principles for this approach are:

**ANALYSING RISK AND PROTECTIVE FACTORS – APPLYING THE KNOWLEDGE TO PROMOTE POSITIVE DEVELOPMENT**

1. Taking a holistic view at different levels:

   a. Child:

      i. health, growth and development,
      ii. behaviour and emotional well-being,
      iii. stable and affectionate social relationships,
      iv. self-efficacy: independence, identity.

   b. Parenting:

      i. meeting needs for care and protection,
      ii. sensitivity and responsive communication and stimulation,
      iii. warmth and affection,
      iv. guidance and boundaries for behaviour.

   c. Family and social environment:

      i. physical and mental health of parents,
      ii. cohesion or chaos in the family functioning,
      iii. amenities (including housing), facilities and income,
      iv. social network and community resources.

2.  Taking an individual view of the child's circumstances. While all children have the same developmental needs, the individual characteristics of the child, e.g. age, sex, temperament and the cultural approach of the family, affect the way these needs are met.

3.  Systematic recording and checking of facts. Facts should be noted in a non-judgemental manner. Assumptions and opinions should be separated from facts. Any differences of opinion regarding the situation and the likely impact on the child of what is happening should be noted.

4.  Considering interactions between various factors, which may provide protection or create further vulnerability.

5.  Working in partnership with the child and the family. Even the most well-meaning practitioners run the risk of alienating the child and/or the family in the process of supporting them. Genuine enquiry, attentive listening, focus on the well-being of the child and a supportive stance, with clarity of one's professional role and responsibilities, help forge a constructive partnership.

6.  Taking steps to do what is required for care and protection of the child, including preventive actions, raising concerns and timely intervention as per the local procedures.

**Further reading**

*In Brief: The Impact of Early Adversity on Children's Development.* www.developingchild.harvard.edu/library/ (accessed 1 June 2013).

Keating, Daniel P. (ed.) (2011) *Nature and Nurture in Early Child Development.* New York: Cambridge University Press.

Shonkoff, J. P. and Phillips, D. A. (eds) (2000) *From Neurons to Neighbourhoods: The Science of Early Child Development.* Washington, DC: National Academy Press.

# Clinical evaluation

# Vision and hearing

Early identification of vision and hearing difficulties is always at the top of the list for practitioners working with children, and for good reasons. First, impairments in these sensory modalities are relatively common and, when significant, can permanently affect a child's development. Second, many of the impairments of hearing and vision are functionally correctable. Although hearing screening programmes, using physiological tests of hearing soon after birth, and orthoptic tests of vision in pre-school children are in place in some countries, including the UK, the imperative of early identification based on concerns, enquiry and observation of visual and hearing behaviour remains.

**VISION**

Tests of vision in children are best performed by trained clinicians, e.g. orthoptists or optometrists. Other practitioners working with children contribute to the early identification of visual impairments through proactive eliciting of concerns, observation of visual behaviour and seeking further specialist examination as required. Poor visual behaviour, the presence of a squint, or abnormal eye movements can be presenting features of a rare but serious eye condition or systemic disorders such as a cataract, glaucoma and retinoblastoma, which are sight- or life-threatening and are treatable.

The most common vision disorders among children are squint, amblyopia and optical problems impairing *visual acuity*. At least 2 per cent of children have amblyopia, a condition of reduced vision in which the eye itself is healthy, but because of a difference between vision in each eye or squint the brain has either suppressed or failed to develop the visual function. It is usually unilateral but rarely may be bilateral. About 1 per cent of infants and 3–7 per cent of young children have a squint.

Visual acuity is rather poor at birth but improves quickly over the next few months, reaching near adult levels by 6–8 months of age. As a major sensory modality, improving vision enables a child to perceive and interact with the social and physical world. Awareness of this changing visual behaviour is useful for eliciting information from parents and making observations.

## Systematic enquiry

The enquiry of parents starts with open-ended questions in order to elicit any concerns:

- Do you have any concerns about your child's vision?
- Is there anything about your child's visual behaviour (the way s/he looks at things) that gives you cause for concern?

This is followed by a more focused age-related enquiry about visual behaviour:

### From 1 week

- Does your baby turn to diffuse light?
- Does your baby stare at your face?

### By 2 months

- Does your baby look at you, follow your face if you move from side to side?
- Does your baby smile responsively back at you?
- Do your baby's eyes move together?

### By 6 months

- Does your baby look around with interest?
- Does your baby try to reach out for small objects?
- Do you think your baby has a *squint*? (Squint is now definitely abnormal, however slight and temporary.)

## By 9 months

- Does your baby poke and rake very small objects such as crumbs or 'hundreds and thousands' cake decorations with fingers?

## By 12 months

- Does your baby point to things he/she wants?
- Does your baby recognise people he/she knows from across the room, before they speak to him/her?

The essential elements of visual examination are given in Table 5.

Equipment required for examination: hundreds and thousands (or other 1–1.5 mm sugar strands); 1-inch cube; ophthalmoscope; small torch.

**Observation/ examination**

*Table 5* Observable visual behaviour.

| | | |
|---|---|---|
| **Response to light** | Blinks to flash and turns to diffuse light | Newborn |
| **Visual fixation** | Fixes and follows near face | 6–8 weeks |
| | Watches adult at 1.5 metres | 4 months |
| | Fixates 1-inch cube at 30 cm | 5 months |
| | Fixates 1.5 mm (hundreds and thousands) at 30 cm | 9 months |
| **Red reflex**[1] | Using an ophthalmoscope | At birth and 6–8 weeks |
| **Abnormal eye movements** | Watching eye movements while the child fixates on an object held in front of the eyes | Birth onwards |
| **Squint**[2] | The corneal reflex test; cover-uncover or alternate-cover test | From 3 months of age |
| **Visual acuity**[2] | Sonksen Silver visual acuity test | From 3 years of age |

[1] To exclude serious conditions, e.g. retinoblastoma and congenital cataract.
[2] Formal tests for pre-school children are best carried out by orthoptists.

**Squint**

A *squint* (strabismus) is a condition where the eyes point in different directions. One eye may turn inwards, outwards, upwards or downwards while the other eye looks forward. Squints are common and affect about 1 in 20 children. They usually develop before a child is 5 years of age but can appear later. Up to around 3 months of age, many babies occasionally squint as their vision develops; however, persistent squint at any age requires an ophthalmological opinion.

The majority of squints are first recognised by parents. The corneal reflex test (Hirschberg test) is performed by shining a light in a person's eyes and observing where the light reflects off the cornea. This light reflex is normally central and symmetrical in both eyes. In divergent squint (exotropia) the light reflection is seen on the medial aspect of the cornea and in convergent squint (esotropia) on the lateral aspect of the cornea (see illustrations). Some squints may not be apparent on such examination and a cover-uncover test can be used by a trained clinician. These tests are not always easy to perform or interpret and a referral to orthoptists should be made if there is any doubt, parental concern or a family history.

*corneal reflex test:*

*a. normal: light reflection on the cornea is central and symmetrical*

*b. in-turning eye, with outward displacement of the light reflection*

Squints can also cause:

1. blurred vision

2. double vision

3. lazy eye (amblyopia) – when the brain starts to ignore signals coming from the eye with the squint.

- Looking at objects closely

- Not responding to carer's expressions; not giving eye contact

- Erratic eye movements

- Poking or rubbing of eyes.

Conductive hearing loss is extremely common. At least half of pre-school children have a history of one or more episodes of 'glue ear', or otitis media with effusion (OME). Persistent OME, which may have adverse effects on children's language and behaviour, affects about 5–10 per cent of children. Parental smoking is a risk factor for children developing OME. Significant sensorineural hearing loss (SNHL), requiring a hearing aid, is present in about 16 per 10,000 children. Delayed identification of children with congenital or acquired hearing loss may result in deficits in speech and language development, poor educational achievement, and behaviour and emotional difficulties.

**HEARING**

It should be checked whether a child has undertaken the neonatal hearing screen and, if missed, a referral should be made. Awareness of risk factors (Box 2) forms the basis for proactive enquiry of parents and for a referral to local audiology services. Tests for hearing (Box 3) require proper training and a suitable testing environment and are best conducted by audiology services. Subjective impressions or poorly done behavioural tests of hearing can cause delay in identification of hearing impairment.

**BOX 2** Risk factors for congenital or acquired hearing loss

- Family history of sensorineural hearing loss

- History of maternal infection during pregnancy, e.g. toxoplasmosis, rubella, herpes, cytomegalovirus and syphilis

- Ear and other craniofacial anomalies

- Hyperbilirubinemia at levels requiring exchange transfusion

- Birthweight less than 1500 grams

- Genetic syndromes known to include SNHL, e.g. Down's syndrome, Waardenburg syndrome

- Childhood disease associated with SNHL, e.g. meningitis, mumps, measles

- Ototoxic medication, e.g. Gentamicin

- Recurrent or persistent OME for at least 3 months

- Head trauma with fracture of temporal bone

- *Neurodegenerative disease*, e.g. Hunter's syndrome, or demyelinating disease, e.g. Friedrich's ataxia, Charcot-Marie-Tooth syndrome.

**Systematic enquiry**

The enquiry of parents is the most important aspect of early identification of hearing impairment in the community. It starts with open-ended questions in order to elicit any concerns:

- Has the child has undertaken the neonatal hearing screen?

- Do you have any concerns about your child's hearing?

- Is there anything about your child's hearing behaviour that gives you a cause for concern?

This is followed by a more focused age-related enquiry about hearing behaviour:

- **From birth**

  - startles or blinks at loud sound

■ **From 1 month**

   ■ quietens to listen to sudden prolonged sound such as a vacuum cleaner

■ **4 months**

   ■ smiles or coos in response to being spoken to

■ **6–7 months**

   ■ turns to locate a person talking

■ **9 months**

   ■ listens attentively and *babbles*

■ **12 months**

   ■ responds to name.

Observing hearing behaviour in a clinic setting:

**Observation/ examination**

■ Children's responses to sounds and conversations are noted. However, such observations are often unreliable due to ambient noise, visual cues or guessing by the child. Behavioural tests of hearing are best conducted in a soundproof room by trained testers.

■ A general practitioner or paediatrician should examine children suspected of having a hearing impairment for signs associated with congenital disorders, e.g. heterochromia of the irises, malformation of the auricle or ear canal, dimpling or skin tags around the auricle, cleft lip or palate, asymmetry or hypoplasia of the facial structures, *microcephaly* and abnormal pigmentation of hair or skin.

> **BOX 3** Tests of hearing in children
>
> **Physiological tests**
>
> These tests are conducted in audiological clinics to measure cochlear/ brainstem responses to sounds:
>
> ■ Evoked or automated otoacoustic emissions.
>
> ■ Automated brainstem responses.
>
> **Behavioural tests**
>
> These tests examine children's response to sounds. They are best conducted in a soundproof clinic by trained testers, using standardised equipment and avoiding visual cues.
>
> ■ Distraction hearing test: at age 7–18 months .
>
> ■ Play audiometry: at age 2–4 years. Child attention span may limit the success of the test.
>
> ■ Conventional *audiometry* (speech and frequency-specific stimuli presented through earphones): from age 3½ years.

**Red-flag signs of possible hearing problems**

■ Lack of response to voices

■ Lack of response to environmental sounds

■ Listening to TV/radio at loud volume

■ Inattentiveness

■ Being unsettled at nursery/school

■ Speech and language problems.

Practitioners should clarify and confirm any concerns from parents and have a low threshold for making a referral to an audiologist or orthoptist/ophthalmologist, as per the local service policy or availability. Children with poor hearing or vision may also require developmental guidance, and early educational advice by specialist teachers, requiring a referral to the local services.

**What to do if there is a concern or abnormal finding on observation/ examination?**

# Self-care and independence

Beginning in the later part of infancy, children start developing independent self-care skills. Cultural and family practices, views about the value of independence in activities of daily living and concerns about safety, at least to some degree, affect what and when children learn about self-care. However, it is useful to enquire about these skills as they relate to the child's general cognitive ability and also provide information about any stresses related to childcare at home.

Children's initial attempts relate to feeding and start with indicating need by grabbing a bottle or a spoon (6 months) and sucking food from a spoon. By 9 months they can hold, bite and chew from food, such as a biscuit or a banana, and can grasp a spoon – only achieving a messy attempt to feed with it by 12 months. At about the same time they can drink from a cup (more effectively by 18 months) and they also start assisting with putting clothes on, e.g. by holding out an arm for a sleeve and a foot for a shoe. By 2 years of age they can feed themselves competently with a spoon and drink from a cup – putting the cup back without spilling. They also now verbalise their toilet needs. Food neophobia (reluctance to try new foods) is common in children between 18 months and 3 years, but can cause carers significant anxiety.

Children begin to use a fork and spoon by the age of 3–3½ years and a knife and fork competently by 5 years. By 3½–4 years they can wash their hands and can undress and dress themselves with little supervision. By 5 years children can usually feed, dress/undress and brush their teeth independently.

Most information regarding self-care skills is gathered on enquiry of parents/carers, although some practitioners will be in contexts that allow direct observation of eating, drinking, dressing and toileting.

The enquiry of parents starts with open-ended questions in order to elicit any concerns:

**Systematic enquiry**

■ Do you have any concerns about your child's feeding, chewing or swallowing?

■ Do you think your child is more or less independent than other children of the same age?

This is followed by more focused age-related enquiry about independence and self-care (Table 6).

*Table 6* Self-care ability.

| Expected age range | |
| --- | --- |
| ■ **Does your baby try to hold a bottle/beaker/mug to drink?** | 6–9 months |
| ■ **Does your baby hold some food such as a biscuit or a banana to eat?** | 8–10 months |
| ■ **Does your baby help in dressing/undressing, e.g. by putting arms up or lifting foot?** | 12–18 months |
| ■ **Does your child feed him/herself with a spoon?** | 15–24 months |
| ■ **Does your child drink from a cup and put it down again without spilling?** | 12–24 months |
| ■ **Can your child eat with a fork and/or a knife?** | 3½–4½ years |
| ■ **How independently can your child dress now?** | Generally independent by 5 years |
| ■ **Can your child wash his/her hands and dry with a towel?** | |
| ■ **Can your child brush his/her teeth independently?** | |
| ■ **Can your child use the toilet independently?** | |

Most of the variation in self-help and independent skills can be attributed to socio-cultural context. However, neurological and developmental disorders affecting general development, perception and movement coordination can result in significant delay or

**Red flags or limit ages – significant delay or abnormality**

specific difficulties, e.g. coughing/choking on swallowing. Further help should be obtained for:

- Any concern regarding the infant's feeding or swallowing
- Lack of interest or ability to feed self beyond the age of 2 years
- Lack of bowel control beyond the age of 3 years
- Rigid insistence on self-imposed routines about self-care, including severely restricted diets.

# Motor development: *birth-1 year*

During infancy children acquire muscle strength, balance and coordination; they lose primitive reflexes and gain protective reflexes; *muscle tone* changes and posture improves. They become independently mobile. The examination of motor development is not simply reliant on milestones of development, but includes qualitative observations of posture, at rest and in movement; any neurological impairment; and information regarding family and birth history.

**Typical developmental pattern**

- Loss of primitive reflexes by 3 months and appearance of protective reflexes (6 months onwards) (Table 7).

- Reducing flexor tone in the limbs resulting in increased range of movements, e.g. *popliteal angle* (see figure, p. 48) 90° at 2 months, 100° at 5 months and 150° at 9 months (Amiel-Tison and Grenier 1986).

- Improving strength, postural control and stability – in *cephalocaudal* direction:

  - head control (3–4 months)

  - trunk stability – straight spine in sitting by 8 months

  - legs – weight bearing ( 6–7 months), standing (9–15 months) (Piek 2006).

- Most children (80 per cent) sit independently between 7 months (mean age) and 11 months (97th centile) and walk between 13 months (mean age) and 18 months (97th centile). About 9 per cent of children do not crawl before walking and shuffle on their bottom, often with a family history of bottom shuffling and/or low *muscle tone*; they are also very late in independent sitting (12 months mean age, 15 months 97th centile) and independent walking (17 months mean age and 24 months 97th centile). There is small group of children (1 per cent) who skip crawling or shuffling altogether and go straight to independent walking, a bit before the rest of their peer group (11 months mean age and 14 months 97th centile). All these three groups have normal patterns. However, a neurological examination is recommended for those who are not walking by 18 months of age to exclude any disorder (Robson 1984).

**Systematic enquiry**

Enquiry of carers starts with open-ended questions:

- Do you have any concerns about the way your baby moves his arms/legs or body?
- Have you ever noticed any odd or unusual movements?
- Has your baby ever seemed too floppy or too stiff?
- Does your baby have a strong preference for one hand and ignore the other hand?
- Are you concerned that the movements on one side are different from the other?

This is followed by more focused age-related enquiry:

- When did your baby start to hold his/her head up?
- When did your baby sit independently?
- How does your baby move around on the floor?
- How does your baby move from one position to the other?

**Red flags from family, birth and medical history**

- Any family history of delayed walking or impaired movements
- Birth or neonatal difficulties
- Feeding, swallowing
- A history of seizure disorder.

Equipment required for examination:
floor mat; visually attractive toy.

Spontaneous posture and movements

| | |
|---|---|
| **Lying on back (supine)** | Movements should be free and symmetrical on both sides. |
| Spontaneous movements of head, arms and legs, and hands | Turns head to visually follow an object by 180° (3 months). |
| | Hands mostly kept open (2 months). |
| | Bringing hands together and to mouth while looking at hands (3 months). |
| | Kicks legs vigorously, alternating or together (3 months). |
| Rolling | Rolling from supine to prone and back (5–7 months). |

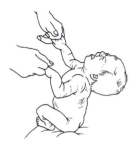

*pull to sit: head lag*

| | |
|---|---|
| **Lying on abdomen (prone)** | Lifts head up 90° and side to side (3 months). |
| Control of head and trunk trunk posture | Lifts chest on arms/hands (4–8 months). |
| | Belly or commando crawling (6–7 months), crawling on hands and knees (8–9 months). |
| **Pull to sit** | Little or no head lag by 3 months. |
| | Braces shoulders and raises head up (5–6 months). |

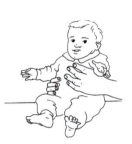

*head control, supported sitting*

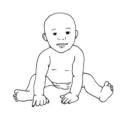

*sitting, hands forward*

| | |
|---|---|
| **Sitting** | Observe head control in supported sitting and spine – straight or curved. |
| | Sitting with (5–6 months) or without (6–8 months) hand support and reaching out with hands to manipulate objects. Pulls self to |

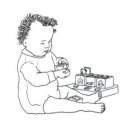

*independent sitting*

|                              |                                                                                     |
|------------------------------|-------------------------------------------------------------------------------------|
|                              | sitting by 9 months and turns around to look and pick up objects.                   |
| **Standing**                 | Observe weight bearing on supported standing and leg posture.                       |
|                              | Pulling to stand (7–12 months) and standing holding to furniture.                   |
|                              | Sits from standing without falling (7–9 months).                                    |
| **Prewalking and walking**   | Crawls/shuffles/rolls.                                                              |
| **Walking**                  | Walks holding to furniture (11–12 months).                                          |
|                              | Takes few steps holding both/ one hand/s (11–12 months) or independently (12–13 months). |

## Examine (eliciting motor behaviour)

The observations of spontaneous movements are made during natural play, encouraging the child to move, pull to stand, cruise, etc. Checking of tone, range of movements and reflexes are part of neuro-motor examination done with the general examination.

*range of movements: popliteal angle*

| | |
|------------------------------|-------------------------------------------------------------|
| **Tone**                     | Any stiffness/floppiness on movement                        |
|                              | Range of movements                                          |
| **Ventral suspension**       | Head control and spine                                      |
| **Primitive reflexes**       | Grasp, Moro, asymmetric tonic neck reflex (Table 7)         |
| **Support or protective reflexes** | Downward, sideward, forward (Table 7)                 |

*Table 7* Primitive and protective/support reflexes.

| | Emerge | Disappear | Eliciting |
|---|---|---|---|
| **Moro** | Birth | 4 months | Elicited by sudden, slight (2.5 centimetres) dropping of the examiner's hand supporting the baby's head. The response consists of symmetrical wide abduction of the arms and opening of the hands. Within moments, the arms come together again, simulating an embrace. |
| **Palmar grasp** | Birth | 3 months | Stroking infant's palm with a finger. |
| **Asymmetric tonic neck reflex (ATNR)** | 2 weeks | 6 months | When the face is turned to one side, the arm and leg on the side to which the face is turned extend and the arm and leg on the opposite side flex. Indicates the possibility of motor disorder if it is persistent or present beyond 6 months. |

*Moro reflex*

*grasp reflex*     *asymmetric tonic neck reflex*

*protective/support reflexes:*

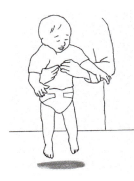

*down*

Protective/support reflexes: These reflexes develop from 4–5 months onwards and can be absent or abnormal in motor disorders

| | | | |
|---|---|---|---|
| **Downward parachute reflex** | 5 months | When held and rapidly lowered the infant extends and abducts both legs, toes pointing down. |
| **Sideward parachute reflex** | 6 months | Infant puts arms out to save if tilted off balance. |
| **Forward parachute reflex** | 7 months | Arms and hands extend on forward descent to ground. |

Source: Heywood and Getchell (2009).

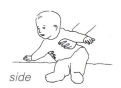

*side*     *forward*

**Atypical patterns**

Children's *muscle tone*, their preferred resting posture in infancy (preferring to lie on tummy or back) and their family history influence motor developmental sequences.

■ Children with atypical pre-walking movement patterns, e.g. bottom shuffling, are late in achieving independent sitting and walking.

■ Preterm infants commonly show early *hypotonia*, increased flexor tone in limbs, extensor *hypertonia* in neck and trunk muscles and poorly coordinated movements. Their motor milestones are often delayed. There are large individual differences in outcomes (Clarke 2005) and follow-up is needed to identify those with lasting impairments.

(Also see Impaired gross motor function in Making sense of findings.)

**Red flags or limit ages – significant delay or abnormality**

■ Fisting of hands beyond 3 months

■ Poor head control at 4 months

■ Persistence of primitive reflexes beyond 6 months

■ Persistence of flexor hypertonia in lower limbs (*popliteal angle* <150° beyond 9 months)

■ Not sitting independently with straight spine by 9 months

■ Not walking independently by 18 months

■ Abnormality of movements

■ persistent repetitive movements

■ asymmetry of movements

■ Abnormality of tone, balance or coordination:

■ undue floppiness or stiffness

■ poor balance

■ poor coordination

- Red flags from general examination:

  - poor eye movements, e.g. *nystagmus*

  - small head circumference

  - dimple, pit or tuft of hair at the bottom of spine suggestive of spina bifida occulta

  - congenital abnormality of hips or feet.

Delayed or abnormal motor development – causes and investigations

**Isla**

Gross motor: Neuro-motor examination

# Motor development: *1-5 years*

From 1 to 5 years children show improvements in control, coordination and balance of their movements. The range of variation in early motor development is substantial. An assessment of motor development should not be over-reliant on milestones of development, but include qualitative observations of posture, at rest and in movement; any associated movements, any neurological impairment and information regarding family and birth history.

**Typical developmental pattern**

After the onset of independent walking, children refine their movement patterns: they develop anticipatory muscle movements and improved coordination and balance as reflected in the following abilities:

- Squat to pick up a toy off the floor (14–18 months).

- Climb into an adult chair to sit (18 months).

- Narrowing of the *walking base* (how far apart legs are kept): at the onset of walking they keep their arms spread out rigidly and legs wide apart (wide base) for better support. The base narrows, with feet only slightly apart at 2 years and in line with body by 4 years.

- Arms move reciprocally with legs by 2 years.

- Toddlers walk with a flat-footed *gait* with some toe walking, particularly when excited or running. They walk mostly with a heel-toe gait about 4–6 months after beginning to walk.

- They can run carefully by 2 years.

- Walk up stairs without holding a support at around 30–36

months (one foot at each step), and walk down stairs between 3 and 4 years of age.

- They can walk a narrow straight line, stand and walk on tiptoes and run around furniture by 3 years.

- Children can throw a ball overhand by 2 years; kick one from 2½ to 3 years and catch a large ball by 3 years.

- They can hop and skip and stand briefly (five seconds) on one foot by 5 years.

Enquiry of parents starts with open-ended questions in order to elicit any concerns:

**Systematic enquiry**

- Do you have any concerns about the way your child moves, walks or runs?

- Have you ever noticed any odd or unusual movements?

- Are you concerned about any unusual stiffness or floppiness of movements?

- Do you think your child's physical skills are in line with other children of the same age?

This is followed by more focused, age-related questions:

- When did your child start to walk independently?

- Can your child run/jump/throw a ball/kick a ball?

- Can your child go up and down stairs? If yes, how?

Equipment required for examination:
floor mat; large ball, small ball; taped line on floor.

**Observation/ examination (or enquire of the carer)**

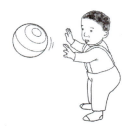

*throwing a ball overhand*

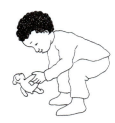

*picking up an object from the floor*

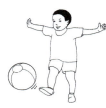

*kicking a ball*

The following activities may be observed, depending on age:

**Walking**
- Pre-walking – crawling/shuffling
- Hand held/independent
- Base of walking – wide/normal
- Running

**Climbing**
- Onto furniture
- Stairs: going up and down steps, with/without support, one or both feet each step

**Jumping**
- Both feet together

**Balance**
- Stable standing
- Stooping to pick up toy off the floor (15–18 months)
- Kicking a large ball
- Throwing a ball overhand
- Standing on one foot for five seconds
- Walking along a line
- Standing on tiptoes
- Hopping/skipping

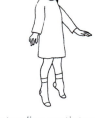

*standing on tiptoe*

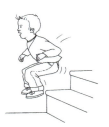

*jumping both feet together*

*coming down stairs: with support*

*coming down stairs independently*

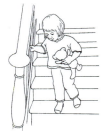

*standing on one foot*

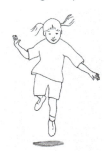

*hopping/skipping*

- The observations of spontaneous movements are made by encouraging the child playfully to walk, run, pick up a toy off the floor, throw, catch, kick, etc.

- Neuro-motor examination is undertaken if there is any concern regarding motor or general development – this must include measurement of head circumference, examination of eyes for any abnormal movements, skin for any abnormal marks, and spine (see Physical examination and investigations, p. 104).

**Examine - eliciting motor behaviour**

The following should prompt further assessment by a physiotherapist and/or a paediatrician:

**Red flags or limit ages - significant delay or abnormality**

- not walking independently by 18 months;

- walking with a narrow *gait* (keeping both legs very close together) at 18 months;

- walking on toes all or most of the time six months after starting to walk or after the age of 3 years;

- still walking with a wide gait (legs too far apart) and with poor balance at 2 years;

- walking or running awkwardly at 3 years;

- unable to climb stairs at 3 years;

- unable to catch, throw or kick a ball at 4 years;

- unable to balance well on one leg at 4 years;

- climbs stairs awkwardly at 5 years;

- any loss or regression of skills (urgent referral for a paediatric opinion should be made);

- any asymmetry of movements – moves arms or legs more or on one side of body;

- any stiffness of movements;

■ any motor delay with associated drooling or difficulty in eating.

Delayed or abnormal motor development – causes and investigations

**Louisa**

Gross motor skills

**Joshua**

Gross motor skills

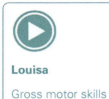

**Alfie**

Gross motor skills

**Further reading**

Heywood, K. M. and, Getchell, N. (2009) *Life Span Motor Development*, 5th edn. Champaign, IL: Human Kinetics.

Piek, J. P. (2006) *Infant Motor Development*. Champaign, IL: Human Kinetics.

Sudgen, D. A. and Wade, M. G. (2013) *Typical and Atypical Motor Development*. London: Wiley.

# Fine motor skills and non-verbal cognition: *birth-1 year*

In early infancy, the effects of improving muscle tone, strength and coordination are apparent in all movements. Improving eye-hand coordination and refinement of movements enable infants to explore the world. At the same time the development of perceptual and non-verbal *cognitive* abilities – mental representation of objects, *working memory* and flexible and sustained attention – also become apparent in many of the infants' activities.

Making sense of the physical world – non-verbal cognition

**Typical developmental pattern**

*Fine motor movements*

■ Increasing coordination of vision with head movement – visual following of a face (6–8 weeks) and of a dangling toy from side to side (3 months). Watching own hand movements (hand regard) (3 months) or objects held in hands (4 months).

■ Improving depth perception and differentiated hand movements – initial two-handed reach is replaced by single-handed reach (5–6 months).

■ Achieving sharp visual focus and differentiation of movements – exploration with index finger 8–9 months.

■ Maturing grasp: improving apposition of tips of finger with the tip of thumb (raking palmar – 6 months, pincer (thumb–finger: 9–10 months) and fingertips (12 months) (see series of illustrations of cube and small object grasps, pp. 59–60).

■ Releasing with pressure on hand or surface (10–11 months); controlled release – puts one cube on top of another (13 months).

*Non-verbal cognition*

- Relating objects together: by banging or clicking them from 6 months, placing things in and out of containers at 9–15 months and inserting pegs into holes by 15 months.

- Cause and effect and means–end concepts: these concepts emerge as simple acts such as shaking of a bell (7 months), using cause-and-effect toys – pressing large buttons to activate a musical toy (9 months), intentional means–end actions such as pulling a toy with a string (9 months) and moving a car (12 months).

- *Permanence of object*: understanding that objects continue to exist even when they are out of view – at 6–8 months infants begin to look for a partially hidden object and between 9 and 10 months they are able to search for a toy which has been completely hidden in their view.

- Categorisation/functional use: use of common objects/toys, e.g. toy car, cup, spoon, bell, telephone (on self/doll/mother). By 10–12 months of age infants use similar-looking objects/toys in the same way, e.g. moving toys that look like a vehicle and by 14 months they show '*definition-by-use*', e.g. using a hairbrush to brush their hair.

**Systematic enquiry**

Enquiry of parents starts with open-ended questions in order to elicit any concerns:

- Do you have any concerns about the way your child uses his/her hands to reach for or to pick up toys or objects?

- Do you have any concerns about the way he/she uses common objects and plays with toys?

- Have you ever noticed any asymmetry of his/her movements?

- Have you noticed any unusual hand movements?

This is followed by more focused, age-related questions:

- Have you noticed any hand preference? Or Is s/he left or right handed?

- How does your child play with toys?

Equipment required for examination:
toy with a string (to dangle/pull along), small toys, pop-up toy, car, cup, plate, spoon, hairbrush, telephone; 1-inch cubes; very small object, e.g. piece of string; small bell with clapper; picture book (robust pages); paper and crayon; cloth (to cover toy).

| | |
|---|---|
| **Hand posture** | Mostly closed (or fisted) or open when awake (2 months) |
| **Holds things put in hands** | Holds briefly and waves it about (3 months), takes to mouth, looks at it (4 months) |
| **Hand regard** | Brings both hands/fingers together, plays with fingers, look at hands (3–4 months) |
| **Reaching with hands: for a toy dangled in front when lying on back, or placed in front when sitting (supported)** | Reaches with both hands (3–4 months)<br><br>Reaches with one hand (5 months) |
| **Grasp** | Raking finger grasp for a very small object or a crumb (6 months) |
| | Picks up a crumb or a piece of string between tips of index finger and thumb (9–10 months) |
| | Picks up a 1-inch cube or a small toy with fingertips (12 months) |
| **Relating/exploring toys/objects** | Passes from hand to hand (6–7 months) |
| | Bangs object on floor/table or two objects together (6 months) |
| | Imitates clicking of two small toys/1-inch cubes (8 months) |

*grasps*

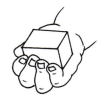

*palmar grasp*

*intermediate grasp*

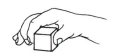

*mature grasp*

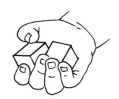

*holds two together*

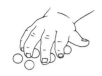

*raking grasp*

*pincer grasp*

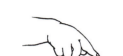

*index finger approach*

*permanence of object:*

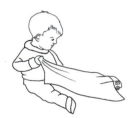

*lifts cloth to find toy*

Holds a toy in hand and explores with the index finger of the other hand, e.g. clapper of a bell (9 months)

Puts cubes in a large cup (10 months)

Releases a small toy to put in on the table, without throwing it, or gives it back (11 months)

Puts one block or a 1-inch cube on top of another (13 months)

**Permanence of object**

**Cause and effect**

**Means–end relationship**

Looks briefly for a toy fallen out of sight

Finds a toy hidden under cloth/paper

Plays with action/pop-up toys

Tries to get a toy out of reach with another object, e.g. a stick or by pulling at a string

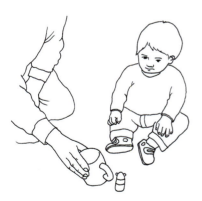
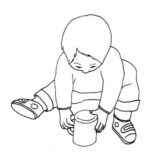
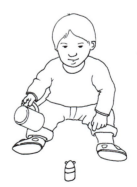

*finds hidden toy*

Fine motor and non-verbal cognitive abilities are best elicited with the use of age-appropriate toys. The objects/toys should be presented to the child one at time or in appropriate combinations, avoiding clutter. A structured approach to presentation helps making of observations. If a child does not show much interest it may be worthwhile to return to that toy/activity later. The child should be comfortably seated, supported if required. Presenter should generate interest and maintain the child's motivation without creating too much excitement; the focus should be kept on the object/activity with suitable praise and encouragement. A brief pause after each step helps in making observations.

**Eliciting responses for observations**

Quality of the activity – how something is done, rather than simply what is done, should be noted. Any partial or emerging response should be noted. The following provides an approach to making these observations; the order can be varied according to the situation.

■ Small (1-inch) cubes/blocks

  ■ Start with presenting one cube by placing it in front of the child on a flat surface or offering it on the flat of your hand (to make it easy to observe the grasp). If the child does not reach for it, place it in his/her hand. Watch what the child does with the cube, e.g. looking, mouthing or hand-to-hand transfer.

  ■ If the child takes one cube, offer another one (note handling of two cubes), and then another one.

  ■ Hold two cubes and click them together encouraging the child to imitate.

  ■ Place a container/cup in front of the child and drop one cube in it, encouraging the child to drop a cube in it and take it out.

  ■ Ask for a cube back by putting open hand out or encourage the child to put the cube on the table. Note release of the cube.

  ■ Place one cube on top of another in front of the child and encourage the child to copy, if the child manages it give more cubes to make a tower.

- Use a bell with a clapper and/or a small object to prompt reach, grasp and exploration.

- Use a toy on a string to check pincer grasp. Place the toy out of reach and string in reach to see means–end relationship (pulling the string to get the toy).

- Use a pop-up or action (cause and effect) toy – observe.

- Use simple toys, e.g. a car, hairbrush, to check functional use.

- Use a simple combination of toys, e.g. cup, spoon, tea pot to observe how the child relates these toys together, uses them functionally on self or offers to examiner/carer or to a doll.

**Red flags or limit ages - significant delay or abnormality**

- Not reaching for a toy placed in front by 6 months

- Not showing interest in exploration of toys/objects by 6 months

- Persistence of 'hand regard' after 9 months

- No index finger exploration by 12 months

- Lack of purposeful use of objects and toys by 12 months

- No cause and effect play by 12 months.

**Isla**

Non-verbal and social development

**Ruby**

Non-verbal and social development

# Fine motor skills and non-verbal cognition: *1-5 years*

After infancy, much of what children do with their hands and fingers – explore, construct, draw and write – reflects development in both fine motor and non-verbal *cognitive* skills – mental representation of objects, *working memory* and flexible and sustained attention. These abilities are observed through activities such as use of day-to-day objects, drawing, bead threading, cutting with scissors, and by using developmental tools of block-construction and shape-sorting/form-boards.

Making sense of the physical world – non-verbal cognition

- Improving bimanual coordination enables children to use one hand to support (e.g. hold) while the other hand acts (e.g. stabilise a toy with one hand and explore with the other) by 18 months.

- Improving dexterity of hands and fingers enables children to turn a door knob and open a screw top by 2 years and cut with scissors, though not yet precisely, by 3 years.

- Better fingertip and hand dexterity is reflected in turning of book pages singly by 2 years; stringing four large beads and holding pencil in a tripod grasp by 3 to 3½ years and doing/undoing large buttons and cutting precisely along a line by 4 years.

**Typical developmental pattern**

*Fine motor movements*

Imitating and copying: children display their understanding of the relationship of objects in space and directionality when they imitate another person making a pattern with blocks or drawing.

When children copy a model that is made out of their view, or shown and removed, they need additional abilities of working memory and recall, planning and rotating objects mentally (see

*Non-verbal cognition*

block structures and copying shape illustrations, p. 67). Imitation, e.g. where the making of the shape or the model is demonstrated for the child, is achieved earlier than the ability to copy from a completed model.

Shape matching, e.g. form-boards: children progress from matching shapes which are easier to rotate in space mentally, such as a circle, to more geometric and irregular shapes. They get better at categorising and visual scanning before matching a shape and stop pushing shapes in wrong holes by 30 months.

Knowledge of colours: observations of children's ability to categorise objects by colour is made by using objects or cards of different colours for naming and matching. By 30 months 50 per cent of children can match cubes/cards by colour. By 42–48 months they can name four colours correctly.

Sorting objects by size: children show a good awareness of size of objects in matching tasks by 30 months. They are able to point to big/small cube/spoon/cup by the age of 3 years and to a l ong/short line drawn on a paper by 42 months (50 per cent) to 54 months (90 per cent).

Drawing: cognitive abilities of left and right orientation, visual attention, working memory and fine motor skills underpin drawing ability. Initial jabbing/stabbing at the paper with some disconnected strokes at 12–15 months reflects a child's exploratory interest and relational understanding.

Scribbling: initially, at 15–18 months, the scribble is a rhythmic back and forth or side to side motion; by 2 years the motion becomes smoother and has circular or wavy appearance. Gradually the drawing becomes more 'contained' and shapely. These drawings may not be visually recognisable but children often name them, showing their representational ability.

Draw-a-man: there is a developmental progression to the 'draw-a-man' task (see Draw-a-man illustrations, p. 67).

Copying shapes: pre-drawn figures (see copying shapes illustrations, p. 67) are presented with a request 'draw one like this one'

– without naming. Any immaturity of figure drawings, e.g. poor closure of shapes and wrong number of angles, is noted.

Enquiry of carers starts with open-ended questions in order to elicit any concerns:

**Systematic enquiry**

- Do you have concerns about the way your child uses his/her hands?

- Do you have concerns about your child's drawing or other constructive play activities?

- Are you concerned about your child's learning?

This is followed by more focused, age-related questions and observations:

- Have you noticed any hand preference? Is your child left or right handed?

- What can your child do with pencil and paper?

- How does your child manage puzzles?

Equipment required for examination:
wooden cubes (six of the same colour); shape-sorter/three-shape form-board; sets of big/small toys, e.g. spoons, cups, cubes; paper and crayons; child scissors; book; shoelaces and large beads; set of matching colour cards and cubes (see Pictures to support examination of verbal and non-verbal skills, p. 144).

**Observation/ examination (or enquire of the carer)**

| | **Book** | Turns pages a few together (18 months)/ (singly 2 years) |
|---|---|---|

*pencil grasps:*

| | **Pencil grasp** | Cylindrical/intermediate/fixed/dynamic tripod |
|---|---|---|

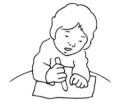

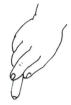

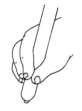

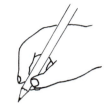

*cylindrical*      *intermediate*      *fixed tripod*      *dynamic tripod*

| | | |
|---|---|---|
| | **Traces along a line** | Trace over a 4-inch long straight line (4 –4½ years) |
| | **Threading large beads** | Threads four large beads with a shoelace (3–3½ years) |
| | **Cutting with scissors** | Tries correctly (may not cut the paper – 3 years)/cuts paper in a straight line (4 years) |
| | **Opening a screw top bottle to take a raisin/penny out** | Opens the bottle/jar to get the raisin/ penny out (22–24 months) |
| | **Handedness** | Mainly uses one hand; use of the other hand to support (18–24 months) |
| | **Using blocks/cubes** | Makes tower (vertical) |
| | | Aligns horizontally |
| | | Makes/copies: a three-brick bridge/train, six-brick stairs (see p. 67 for age norms) |
| | **Drawing** | Makes a mark, scribbles – linear/circular, copies a line, shapes and people (see p. 67 for age norms) |
| | **Shape matching** | Completes three shapes (circle, triangle and square) form-board with visual scanning before putting the shape in by 30 months and six or more shapes by 3 years. |

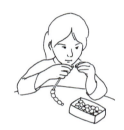

*threads beads*

*shape-matching: form-board*

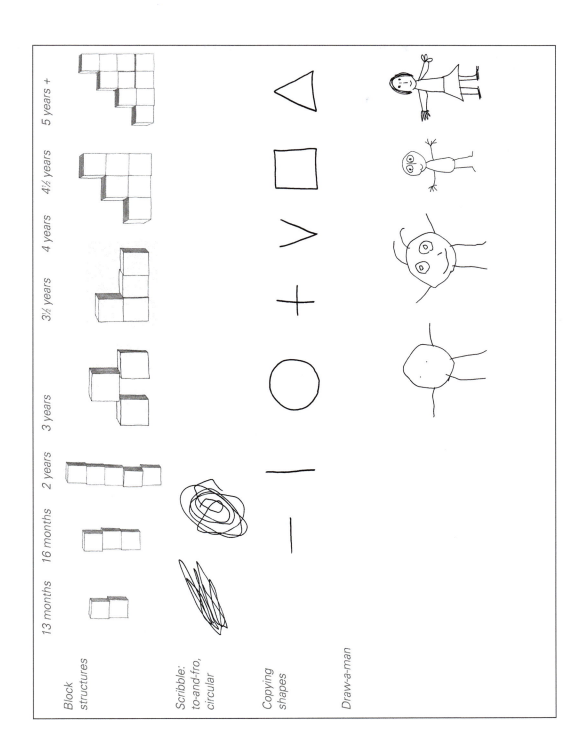

**Eliciting responses for observations**

- Observations of fine motor skills are often made during an informal play session and throughout the observation period. Note is made of any coordination difficulties, tremors or any associated or abnormal movements.

- Structured presentation is required for observing non-verbal cognitive abilities. One task is presented at a time, in the order of increasing difficulty.

- In block building tasks, the child is first encouraged to copy from a model or a drawing. This is done by the examiner using a sheet of paper to hide the model being built and/or by using pre-drawn shapes.

- If the child is unable to copy or follow instructions the examiner makes it easier by showing how it is done – a note is made of the help needed.

- Form-boards or jig-saw puzzles are presented first for simple circle shapes before two or three shape combinations. A three-shape form-board, once completed, is reversed and the child is asked to do it again.

- Tasks are presented in the midline. Sometimes alternating the placing of a crayon, pencil or blocks on each side of the child helps in establishing handedness.

- In addition to the completion of a task, the child's *attention* to task and ways of approaching and responding to a difficult task are noted.

- At all times the focus is kept on the task by removing distractions, keeping the 'chat' to a minimum and encouraging the child with praise. Motivation is maintained by presenting tasks swiftly and creating interest in each new task.

**Red flags or limit ages - significant delay or abnormality**

Poor performance on non-verbal tasks may relate to developmental impairment but may also be due to poor motivation, poor vision and/or hearing, and in some cases, lack of stimulation. Further assessment is indicated for:

- poor fine motor coordination, tremors or associated movements;

- poor following of instructions, poor attention to completion of task, high level of distractibility and generally high level of motor activity;

- inability to stack two blocks with a mature release by 2 years;

- inability to hold a crayon/pencil to make a mark on the paper by 18 months, scribble by 2 years and copy a circle by 4 years;

- generally non-compliant behaviour;

- significant underachievement at any individual task or mild– moderate underachievement across all tasks.

**Louisa**

Non-verbal and social development

**Joshua**

Non-verbal and social development

**Alfie**

Non-verbal and social development

# Speech, language and communication: *birth-1 year*

During infancy the foundations for speech, language and communication are developed through interaction with caregivers. Before speech develops the majority of children are highly competent communicators, able to initiate, maintain and terminate mutually rewarding communicative exchanges. Through non-verbal strategies basic communication functions, such as attracting attention, greeting, requesting, commenting and seeking information, are all within the repertoire of typically developing infants. By 12 months children have the basic motor competencies for speech production, and are able to produce a range of speech sounds, pitch and volume changes and use these to engage in vocal play both alone, and with caregivers. The development of communication is inextricably linked with social behaviour and play.

Theories of language development

## Typical developmental pattern

*Language understanding*

The typical steps to the development of speech, language and communication are:

- Turns to the sound of a soothing human voice (1 month).

- Makes pre-speech lip and tongue movements in response to carer's talk (1 month).

- May appear less responsive to interaction when starts to attend to objects (5 months).

Speech development

- Turns to familiar voices, even when the adult is not in view (6 months).

- Responds when name is called (8 months).

- Understands 'no!' and 'bye bye' (9 months).

- Shows understanding of familiar words for familiar people or embedded in familiar routines, e.g. 'bedtime', 'where's daddy?' (12 months).

- Utters *guttural sounds* when content (1 month).

- Vocalises delightedly in response to chat or enjoyable play with carers (2–3 months).

- Sing-song vowels, single- and double-syllable sounds, e.g. 'goo', 'dada', 'der' to self and others (6 months).

- Imitates playful vocalisations and actions, e.g. cough, smacking lips (9 months).

- *Jargon* – tuneful *babble* with phrase-like intonation (10 months).

- A few consistent 'words', intelligible to familiar carers (12 months).

- Shows clear like, dislike, acceptance and rejection of experiences (6 months).

- Invites adults and other children to interact by vocalising, flapping hands, etc. (8 months).

- Makes requests by pointing (10 months).

Enquiry of carers starts with open-ended questions in order to elicit any concerns:

- Do you have any concerns about your child's communication?

- Do you have any concerns about the sounds your child makes?

- Do you have any concerns about how your baby responds when you talk to him/her?

This is followed by more focused, age-related questions:

- How do you attract your baby's attention?

- How easy is it to direct your baby's attention to things in the environment, e.g. pointing out a dog?

- What words are you sure your baby understands? How do you know?

- Does your baby look at familiar people or objects when you name them?

- What instructions will your baby follow?

- What sounds do you hear your baby making?

- Does your baby have any recognisable words? Would they be understood by people outside the family?

- What languages are spoken in the home? Do you think your baby responds differently to the different languages?

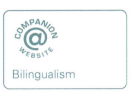

Bilingualism

**Observation/ examination (or enquire of the carer)**

Equipment required for examination:
rattles/bells, bunch of keys, teething toys, telephone, push-along car/train, baby doll/teddy, small cup and spoon, wind-up music box, cloth (for peek-a-boo), wooden bricks, bubbles.

| | |
|---|---|
| **Attention to speech** | Speak to the baby from approx. 2 feet away, in a friendly tone. |
| **Anticipation** | 'I'm coming to tickle you', with friendly facial expression. |
| **Responds to name** | Call name when the baby is engaged in play with a toy. |
| **Responds to tone of voice** | As the baby reaches for a toy, interrupt with a firm 'no!', immediately followed by reassurance. |

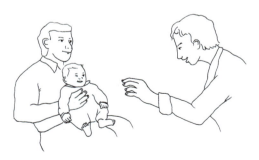

*tickling game (sitting on carer's lap)*

| | |
|---|---|
| **Joint attention** | Shifts attention between a speaker and toys to establish shared focus with communication partner. |
| **Follows simple instructions with cues** | 'Give me the keys [or whatever the baby is holding]' whilst holding out a hand to receive the object (some families use the word 'ta'). |
| | Invite baby to 'clap hands', whilst clapping, with expectant facial expression. |
| **Responds to name \*** | Call name when baby is looking elsewhere but not completely absorbed in play. |
| **Follows a point \*** | Call name, then say 'look' and point to object in middle distance. |
| **Requesting** | Place attractive toy just out of reach. Observe strategies used to request, e.g. reaching, pointing, looking between object and adult. |
| **Gestures** | Does the child wave and say 'bye' on leaving the room in response to a farewell? |

*These items also appear in Social behaviour and play, pp. 85–7.

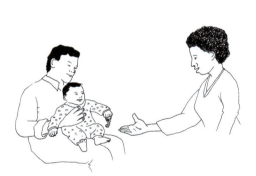
*'give me' + outstretched hand*

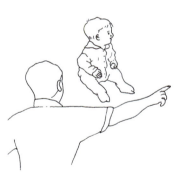
*following a point*

**Eliciting responses for observations**

Much of the assessment of young infants takes place through observation of interaction with familiar caregivers. The examiner then guides the child through the following set of activities:

- Provide age-appropriate toys and ask the carer to 'show me how you would play together with this toy' – observe focus of the baby's attention and response to the carer's speech.

- Having the baby sitting on the carer's lap, facing forwards towards the examiner, but able to access toys on a table top, is an appropriate position to assess response to name, ability to follow instructions with cues, and requesting.

- Encourage the child to make a choice, or to ask for more, by starting and pausing activities, such as blowing bubbles or using a wind-up musical box.

- Observe how the infant references the carer – does he/she share pleasure in activities, or check out the carer's reactions?

- If the child is reluctant to engage with the examiner many activities can be carried out by the carer, under the guidance of the examiner.

**Red flags or limit ages - significant delay or abnormality**

- Not smiling when spoken to by 3 months

- No sounds other than crying by 6 months

- Not recognising own name by 9 months

- Not producing tuneful *babble* by 12 months

- Not showing recognition of any object names by 12 months

- No waving, pointing or other gesture by 12 months.

**Isla**

Social communication and play

**Ruby**

Social communication and play

# Speech, language and communication: *1-5 years*

Language is crucial for the initiation and maintenance of social relationships, for expressing ideas about the world, for thinking and for accessing formal learning. As a foundation life skill, the development of communication has implications for literacy, school performance and employment prospects, as well as a child's well-being and ability to fit in with the family, and wider society.

Speech, language and communication include children's understanding of language, the ability to express themselves through grammatical sentences and clear speech, and the use of non-verbal communication. Communication functions that have been primarily non-verbal become expressed through spoken language of increasing complexity. Between the ages of 1 and 5 years, children make progress in the sophistication of their communication across a range of functions, including:

**Typical developmental pattern**

- controlling the behaviour of others;
- requesting;
- engaging others in interaction, including greetings, farewells, use of names, polite language;
- labelling internal states/emotions (self and others);
- seeking information;
- giving information;
- use of language for pretending and *make-believe*;
- teasing and humour.

The typical steps to the development of speech, language and communication are:

**Language understanding**

■ Understands names of familiar people or objects, embedded in familiar routines, e.g. 'where's your cup?' (12 months).

■ Follows simple commands in *context*, e.g. 'come here', 'give it to me' (12–15 months).

■ Can point to body parts (12–18 months).

■ Selects a named object when other options are available, e.g. 'where's the spoon?' (18 months).

■ Follows two-part instructions, e.g. 'get your cup from the bag' (18–24 months).

■ Picks out objects by function, e.g. 'which one do we drink from?' (24–30 months).

■ Understands sentences of three information-carrying words (ICW), e.g. 'put the cup and the plate on the chair' at 3 years, four ICW at 4 years and five ICW at 5 years.

■ Understands time and sequence concepts, e.g. 'first', 'then', 'last', at 5 years.

**Expressive skills**

■ A few consistent 'words', in amongst *jargon*, at 12 months (intelligible to familiar carers).

■ Rapid increase in vocabulary, single words can be used for a range of reasons – requests, comments, questions (15–18 months). Copies words.

■ Combines two words, e.g. 'doggy gone' (18–24 months).

■ Uses 'no' or 'not' in phrases, e.g. 'no shoes!' (24 months).

■ Refers to past/future events (24 months).

■ Three-word phrases, e.g. 'kick big ball' (30–36 months).

■ Uses pronouns 'I', 'me' , 'you' (24–36 months), followed by 's/he', 'they' (36–40 months).

- Immature grammar (30–48 months), with mastery of adult grammar, with occasional immaturities, by 60 months.

- Most speech sounds are clear by 5 years.

**Verbal cognition**

- Asks questions – 'what's that?' (24 months), 'where . . .?' (30–36 months), 'why?' (36–42 months).

- Can give own name (30 months), sex (36 months), age (48 months), birthday and address (60 months).

- Uses descriptive concepts – big/little, wet/dry, up/down, hot/cold, etc. (from 30–36 months).

- Understands prepositions – in/out/on/off/out of/under/behind, etc. (24–36 months).

- Rote counts, without number concept beyond 1 or 2 (36 months), counting objects 1–5 (40–54 months).

- Recognises named colours (36 months), names colours (42–48 months).

- Understands and uses words to represent categories, e.g. toys, food (42–48 months).

- Uses language to pretend, e.g. 'you be the baby . . .' (42–48 months).

- Enjoys jokes and verbal incongruities, including awareness of rude words (48–60 months).

- Links ideas linguistically – initially using 'and' and 'then' (36–42 months) before 'because' (42–48 months).

- Uses language to compare, e.g. bigger, heavier, strongest (54–60 months).

- Uses of abstract linguistic concepts for temporal sequences 'when . . . then . . .', 'if . . . then . . .' by 5 years.

**Systematic enquiry**

Enquiry of parents begins with open-ended questions in order to elicit any concerns:

- Do you have any concerns about your child's understanding?

- Do you have any concerns about how your child is developing speech?

- Do you have any concerns about how your child is putting sentences together?

This is followed by more focused, age-related questions:

- Can your child point to pictures in a book when you name them?

- Can your child name pictures in books?

- Give me some examples of the words your child uses every day?

- Give me some examples of the phrases your child uses frequently?

- Can everyone understand your child's speech?

- Can you have a conversation with your child? Give me some examples.

- Can your child answer 'where is . . .' questions?

- What sort of questions does your child ask?

- Can your child listen to stories?

- Does your child join in with telling familiar stories?

- How does your child tell you about things that happened when you were not there?

- Can your child give an explanation in response to 'why . . .?' questions?

- What languages are spoken in the home? Do you think your child has similar skills in the different languages?

Equipment required for examination:
doll/teddy, cup, ball, spoon, sock; cubes (different colours – two each of red, blue, green, yellow, orange), large and small cubes; boxes (big and small), plastic animals, e.g. cow, horse, elephant, lion; picture book, with simple narrative (see Pictures to support examination of non-verbal and verbal skills, p. 144).

R – receptive/E – expressive

| | |
|---|---|
| **Points to body parts** | Use a teddy in a game – 'he's coming to tickle your nose – where's your nose?' or ask the child to 'tickle teddy's nose', etc., or use picture of the dog (see Pictures to support examination of verbal and non-verbal skills). |
| **Selects/names objects** | Put out four common objects, e.g. cup, spoon, ball, sock. |
| | R – 'show me/look at/give me the . . .' (18 months) |
| | Wait for eye contact before delivering request, and avoid looking at the named object. |
| | E – 'what is this?' |

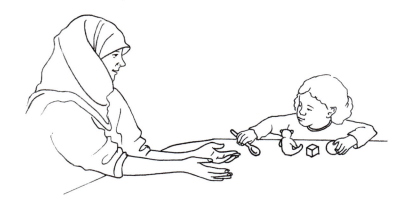

*gives objects on request*

| | |
|---|---|
| **Follows/uses common action words** | With teddy: |
| | R – 'make teddy jump/lie down/drink'<br>E – 'what's teddy doing?' |
| | With pictures (from 24 months): |
| | R – 'which one is drinking/ sleeping, etc?'<br>E – 'what's this girl doing?' |
| **Selects objects by function** | Put out four common objects/pictures, e.g. cup, spoon, ball, sock. |
| | R – 'which one can we kick/wear/drink from?'<br>E – 'what do you do with a sock?' |
| **Follows instructions with concepts** | Using variety of coloured bricks and a box |
| | *Spatial:* |
| | R – 'put the brick in/on/under/behind the box' (in/on – 24–30 months, under/behind 30–36 months). |
| | *Colour:* |
| | R – 'where's the red/yellow/blue/green brick?' (36–40 months) |
| | E – naming four colours (42 months) |
| | The ability to match colours emerges before recognition/naming (30 months) |
| | *Size:* |
| | R – 'put the bricks in the big/little box' (30–36 months) |
| | R – 'show me the long/short line of bricks' (42 months) |
| | R – 'which is the heavier (not larger) brick?' (48 months) |
| | In order to maintain a child's interest it may be necessary to give the instructions via a toy, or have the child manipulate a toy to carry out the instructions. |

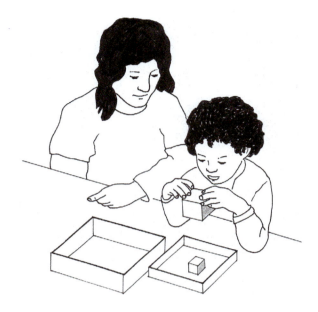

*assessing understanding of concepts: size*

**Follows sentences of increasing length**

Using sets of toys, e.g. animals and small plates

R – 'the <u>cow</u> and the <u>horse</u> want to <u>eat</u>' – three ICW (3 years)

R – 'the <u>elephant</u> and the <u>lion</u> want to <u>dance</u> and <u>jump</u>' – four ICW (4–5 years)

E – 'what happened to the elephant?'

there should be an alternative for each underlined word.

**Uses language to tell a simple narrative**

Using a simple story book (with few printed words) or a set of miniature toys – start to tell a simple story and then ask the child to take over 'now you tell me what's happening' – observe sentence length and use of *concept vocabulary*.

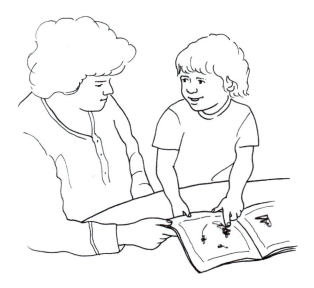

*telling a simple story*

| | |
|---|---|
| **Describing past events** | Ask the child to tell you about a recent event (holiday, party, etc.) – observe sentence structure, ability to produce a coherent narrative and accommodate to the listener's knowledge of the topic. |
| **Giving explanations** | Ask the child questions about the purpose of common objects, e.g. 'what is a spoon for?', 'why do we wear shoes?' |
| **Answers hypothetical questions** | Ask 'what would you do if you were hungry/cold?', etc. |

**Eliciting responses for observations**

A semi-structured play session is useful for gathering information about the child's speech, language and communication, alongside social interaction and play skills (see Social behaviour and play – 1–5 years: Eliciting responses for observations, p. 92). Such a session usually begins with 'free play' with some developmentally appropriate toys, e.g. cause-and-effect and construction toys and/

or a doll/family/tea set and/or action figures. The examiner than guides the child through the following set of activities:

- Interactive play activities to observe turn-taking and imaginative play.

- Setting up *pretend play* and role play activities to check the child's creativity, and use of language to negotiate.

- Free play can be a springboard for to-and-fro conversations about the child's own experiences, e.g. 'what toys do you like to play with at home?', 'who do you like to play with?', etc.

- Table-top activities to assess levels of language understanding (see above) should be attempted only after the child is comfortable in joint free play.

- If the child is reluctant to engage with the examiner many activities can be carried out by the carer, under guidance from the examiner.

**Red flags or limit ages – significant delay or abnormality**

- Not responding to familiar songs and rhymes by 18 months

- Unable to follow simple commands in routines by 18 months

- No recognisable words by 18 months

- Not joining words together by 24 months

- Not using three-word phrases routinely by 36 months

- Speech is largely unintelligible to unfamiliar listeners by 36 months

- Language consists mainly of phrases learned from DVDs, with little spontaneous language, at any age

- Unable to understand/use descriptive concept vocabulary (size, position, quantity) by 42 months

- Unable to relate a past event to a listener who was not present by 4 years

- Unable to answer 'where/who . . .' questions by 4 years

- Stammering – blocking or repetition of parts of words by 4 years (brief periods of non-fluency are typical in 3 year olds)

- Unable to hold a coherent conversation or provide reasonably logical responses to questions at 5 years

- Loss of language skills at any age should trigger immediate investigation

**Louisa**

Social communication and play

**Joshua**

Social communication and play

**Alfie**

Social communication and play

# Social behaviour and play:
## *birth–1 year*

COMPANION @ WEBSITE

Development of
social cognition

COMPANION @ WEBSITE

Development of
joint attention

Social behaviour and play underpin future speech, language, communication and cognitive skills. Development in these areas is facilitated through social interaction with carers, and extends to others as the child's social environment broadens. The concept of 'play' has different meanings across cultures; therefore sensitivity may be required when discussing this domain with carers.

**Typical developmental pattern**

- Developing social responsiveness and anticipation.

  - Preference for attending to people/mother (soon after birth).

  - *Social smile* (6–8 weeks).

  - Interactive imitation of smiles, facial expressions and sounds (6–8 weeks).

  - Responds to social games such as peek-a-boo and shows anticipation (6 months).

- Developing *joint attention* (a crucial step for the development of language and communication skills).

  - Follows others' finger point to look at an object (8 months).

  - Uses finger and eye pointing to direct others' attention to share interest (9–12 months).

- Becoming stranger-aware – reacting by withdrawing or crying (7–8 months).

- *Social referencing* – checking back by looking towards the care-giver in new situations (12 months).

- Exploration of toys and objects: looking closely, touching, mouthing and banging (5–6 months)

- Playing with pop-up and action toys with emerging under-standing of cause-and-effect (8–9 months).

- Functional use of toys and objects, e.g. 'talking' on the phone and putting a hat on self (12 months) and on others, e.g. doll, mother (15 months).

**Systematic enquiry**

Enquiry of carers starts with open-ended questions in order to elicit any concerns:

- Do you have any concerns about the way your baby responds to you and to others?

- Do you have any concerns about the way your baby plays with toys?

This is followed by more focused, age-related questions:

- How does your baby respond to you when you smile at him/her?

- Does your baby play nursery games such as pat-a-cake or peek-a-boo with you?

- Does your baby get your attention to show you something?

- How does your baby react to another person not known to him/her?

- What toys does your baby like to play with?

**Observation/ examination (or enquire of the carer)**

Equipment required for examination:
cup, spoon, plate, hairbrush, telephone, car; cloth (for peek-a-boo), pop-up toys; toys that can be safely mouthed.

| | |
|---|---|
| **Social smile** | In response to carer's smile or vocalisation |
| **To-and-fro interactions** | Responsive expressions and sounds in interactions |
| **Social anticipation** | Eager participation in pat-a-cake or peek-a-boo |
| **Follows a point*** | Call name, then say 'look' and point to object in middle distance |
| **Pointing** | ■ To ask<br>■ To share interest |
| **Social referencing** | Checks back with the carer by looking back |
| **Response to name*** | Turns to look |
| **Follows simple directions** | Responds appropriately to 'come' and 'no' |
| **Functional use of toys** | Uses a toy car as a car to make it move; uses a phone, hairbrush, spoon or cup on self or on carer or a doll/teddy |

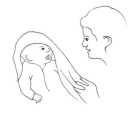

*playing peek-a-boo*

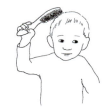

*use of a hairbrush on self*

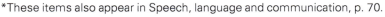

*These items also appear in Speech, language and communication, p. 70.

**Eliciting responses for observations**

■ Social behaviour is observed through participation in various playful activities undertaken during the assessment.

■ Response to name should be elicited from the side at a little distance.

■ The use of day-to-day objects, e.g. cup, spoon, phone, can be modelled to generate interest.

■ The mother/carer should be asked to interact with the infant playfully if there is marked *stranger wariness*.

**Red flags or limit ages - significant delay or abnormality**

A lack of social responsiveness and play skills may be related to poor vision or hearing.

■ Not responding to carer's interactions such as smiles by 8 weeks

- No joyful engagement in fun activities by 5 months
- Lack of visual regard of hands or toys by 5 months
- Lack of interest in toys
- Lack of interest in social games by 9 months
- Excessive mouthing persisting beyond 12 months
- No pointing to make requests or other gestures by 12 months
- No pointing to share interest by 18 months.

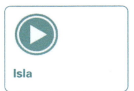

Isla

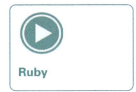

Ruby

*Link here to full videos*

# Social behaviour and play:
## *1-5 years*

Social behaviour includes children's emerging understanding of intentions, desires, feelings and beliefs and how these influence the actions of self and others. It helps them initiate and maintain social relationships and learn in social settings.

The typical steps to the development of social understanding and behaviour in children after infancy are:

■ Activities become more intentional and purposeful by 12 months.

■ Developing a sense of self – recognising self in the mirror (20 months) and in photos (24 months).

■ Expressing self-conscious emotions such as shame and embarrassment (18–24 months).

■ Expressing emotions in words from 2 years.

■ Learning to express emotions appropriately to situations from 3 years.

■ Understanding others' intentions by 10–12 months.

■ Sharing own interest and intention with others through *joint attention* from 12 months.

■ Attributing desires, but not beliefs, to self and others; understanding that these desires may differ from their own, and being able to make connection between desires and positive or negative emotions, e.g. fulfilment of desires leads to positive emotions (from 24 months) (Wellman 2004; Paulin-Dubois *et al.* 2009).

**Typical developmental pattern**

*Becoming self-aware*

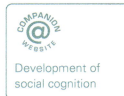

Development of social cognition

*Becoming social*

- Understanding that others think and act on what they believe to be true and that such beliefs may be different for different people (from 2½ to 3 years).

- Understanding that others' beliefs may not be true – *false belief* understanding (4 years).

- Responding to others' expressions of distress by offering some comfort from 2½ years.

- Beginning to share with the peer group from 3 years.

- Negotiating with others to maintain social interactions 4–5 years.

**Social imaginative play**

- Playing with intention, goal and at least a brief plan from 12 months.

- Using common objects in a functional manner, first on self (12 months) and then with carers from 14–18 months.

- Early *pretend play*: acting out familiar routines from 18 months to 2 years.

- Acting out roles and making short sequences of imaginary play acts substituting objects, e.g. a box for a car, from 2½ to 3 years.

- Creating fantasy scenarios using miniature toys or replacement objects from 4 years.

- Following rules cooperatively with other children for group games from 5 years.

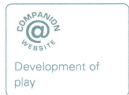

Development of play

**Systematic enquiry**

Enquiry of carers starts with open-ended questions in order to elicit any concerns:

- Do you have any concerns about the way your child responds to you and other people?

- Do you have any concerns about the way your child plays with toys?

- Are there any difficulties in getting eye contact with your child?

This is followed by more focused, age-related questions:

- Does your child ever bring any items of interest, e.g. a drawing or a toy, to show to you?
- How does your child occupy him/herself at home?
- How does your child interact with other children?
- Does your child engage in pretend play (e.g. feeding a doll or teddy, putting a toy in truck and pretending to drive it along)?
- Do you see your child making up stories with toys/action figures?

Equipment required for examination:
telephone, hairbrush, miniatures – dolls, animals, action figures, doll's house furniture, tea set; cause-and-effect toys; construction toys, e.g. Duplo, cubes, string, small pieces of cloth; action figures, unrelated small toys.

**Observation/ examination (or enquire of the carer)**

| | |
|---|---|
| **Social smile** | In response to carer's smile or vocalisation |
| **Social anticipation** | Eager participation in chasing and turn-taking games |
| **Pointing** | ■ To ask<br>■ To share interest |
| **Social referencing** | Checks back with the carer for reassurance |
| **Showing** | Obtains attention of carers/adults to show things to them |
| **Social interactions** | Shows interest in other children. Initiates interactions by getting attention and responds to others. Combines eye contact, facial expressions, gestures and words/sounds to interact. |
| **Group activities** | Joins in some group/shared activities with others |

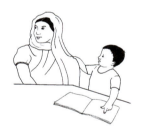

*pointing to show – near object*

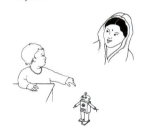

*pointing to show – distant object*

| | |
|---|---|
| **Pretence** | Pretends that objects are something else in play or offers pretend food/drink |
| **Play** | Play in an interactive, turn-taking way with others |

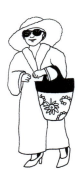

*role play dressing up*

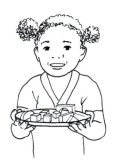

*pretend play – substitution*

**Eliciting responses for observations**

A semi-structured play session is useful for gathering information about the child's social interaction and play abilities, as well as speech, language and communication. Such a session usually begins with 'free play' with some developmentally appropriate toys, e.g. cause-and-effect and construction toys and/or a doll/family/tea set and/or action figures. The examiner then guides the child through the following set of activities:

■ interactive play activities to observe turn-taking and imaginative play;

■ encouraging the child to make a choice, or to ask for more, by starting and pausing activities, such as blowing balloons or bubbles;

■ setting up pretend play and role play activities to check the child's creativity;

■ using play situations for to-and-fro conversations.

If the child is reluctant to engage with the examiner many activities can be carried out by the carer, under guidance from the examiner.

- No pointing or other gesture by 12 months

- No *joint attention* (following a point, and pointing for interest) by 18 months

- Lack of showing with toys or other objects by 18 months

- Absence of simple pretend play (e.g. feeding doll) by 24 months

- Repetitive play with toys (e.g. lining up objects)

- Solitary play with a lack of social interest in others

- Odd approaches to other children or adults

- Minimal recognition or responsiveness to other people's happiness or distress

- Limited variety of imaginative play, especially a lack of social imagination (not joining with others in shared imaginary games)

- Repetitive and persistent acting out of scenes from videos

- Odd relationships with adults (inappropriately friendly/disinhibited or ignores).

**Red flags or limit ages - significant delay or abnormality**

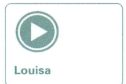

Louisa

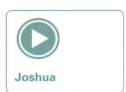

Joshua

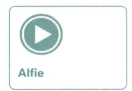

Alfie

*Link here to full videos*

# Attention, impulsivity and activity level

The ability to pay *attention* to tasks and events is essential for learning. Difficulties in paying attention or maintaining attention to tasks is often the reason for children's poor social and educational participation, but sometimes learning difficulties can be the cause of poor attention. *Impulsivity* and high activity levels associated with poor attention may indicate the presence of a disorder, e.g. Attention Deficit Hyperactivity Disorder (ADHD). Enquiry of carers and teachers and observations of attention and behaviour are helpful in making sense of a child's performance and in deciding when further help is needed.

**Typical developmental pattern – attention**

- Birth to 18 months: Infants sustain attention in exploring toys by 5 months and, by 9–12 months, show sustained purposeful activities, correcting errors in looking for hidden objects. However, they are easily distracted towards a dominant stimulus.

- 18 months to 3 years: Children become able to undertake planned sequential activities of increasing complexity, such as matching of shapes/forms, with sustained attention and get better at inhibiting their impulsivity. They, however, remain somewhat resistant to interference and need adult help in shifting their attention to a different task.

- 3–4 years: Attention now becomes more flexible – easily shifting between tasks; selective – able to ignore irrelevant stimuli, and sustained (36 months).

- 4–5 years: Children now voluntarily ignore stimuli which are irrelevant to the task, controlling their focus of attention. They sustain attention to sort objects, such as cards, on two dimensions, e.g. colour and shape.

■ By 5 years of age children integrate information from different sources, e.g. listening to directions without losing focus on the task. They can now make a plan and carry it out with sustained and flexible attention.

Onset and duration of concerns regarding attention are important to note as transient problems often arise due to change of social or physical circumstances, e.g. change of house, ill health or other changes in family dynamics. Although behavioural concerns are often reported from infancy onwards, concerns specifically regarding attention usually start after the age of 4 years. Information from multiple informants across different settings is useful in determining the type of problem and its functional impact.

**Systematic enquiry**

Enquiry of carers starts with open-ended questions in order to elicit any concerns:

■ Do you have any concerns about your child's ability to listen?

■ Are you concerned about your child's activity levels?

■ Can your child quieten down when told s/he is too loud and noisy?

■ Do you think your child's activity levels are affecting learning, family life or interactions with peers?

This is followed by more focused, age-related questions:

■ How long can your child concentrate on activities such as mealtimes, watching TV, listening to stories?

■ Can your child complete simple tasks without becoming distracted?

■ Does your child frequently interrupt without letting others finish what they are saying?

■ Can your child wait for his/her turn?

■ Does your child fidget or squirm a lot?

■ Can your child work in a group?

**Observation/ examination (or enquire of the carer)**

■ Observations are made within activities outlined in previous sections (Fine motor, Speech language and communication, etc.).

■ Direct observations of children's attentional behaviour, *impulsivity*, activity level and function are useful for a number of reasons: first, it helps to put the child's performance on developmental tasks in context, and second, it provides separate observer information, which may not be available for some children who are not yet attending a nursery/school.

■ Observations of attention, like those of emotions and behaviour, should be made across different tasks/activities and over time before making any valid interpretation.

■ Observations across a range of structured tasks (verbal and non-verbal) and unstructured activities, e.g. free play or drawing, also provide information regarding any likely difficulty with a particular domain of development (e.g. poor language understanding) underlying attention difficulties.

■ Clinic-based observations are often affected by the child's anxiety and motivational level and may not be reflective of the child's actual behaviour.

| *Attention and its correlates* | *Observable behaviours* |
|---|---|
| **Listening attention** | ■ Ability to listen to directions fully.<br>■ Listening to directions without losing focus on the task. |
| **Sustained attention** | ■ Ability to stay with and complete purposeful and planned activities. |
| **Distractibility** | ■ Ability to avoid distractions such as other irrelevant objects or activities in the middle of doing a planned task. |
| **Shifting attention** | ■ Any shift in attention with time or with change of activity. |
| **Impulsivity** | ■ Blurting out comments, interrupting others, snatching from the hands, rushing from one object to another. |

| **Activity level** | ■ Increased motor activity – running, climbing or jumping while being required to stay on task. |
| | ■ Too much or loud talking. |
| **Fidgetiness** | ■ Irrelevant movements of hands/legs/feet (e.g. tapping/shaking). |
| | ■ Squirming on the seat, slouching, clowning. |

## Poor attention – clinical and management considerations

■ Concerns about a child's attention become significant when they affect his/her functioning with the family, peer group or school.

■ An underlying disorder, e.g. ADHD, is likely if there are persistent difficulties in a number of features and correlates of attention (described above), in a number of settings, as described by parents, teachers and other professionals/carers.

■ A variety of medical conditions are associated with attention problems in pre-schoolers, including epilepsy, hypothyroidism, low birthweight, hearing loss, and prenatal exposure to teratogens (e.g. foetal alcohol syndrome).

■ Behavioural difficulties, language impairment, social communication difficulties and coordination difficulties are common in children with deficits of attention.

■ A child with significant concerns regarding attention requires further assessment by a paediatrician/child psychiatrist and often needs help from a teacher and psychologist.

Helping children with attention difficulties

■ Parents should be offered help regarding management of their child's behaviour and the development of his/her attentional abilities.

## Further reading

'ADHD: Clinical Practice Guideline for the Diagnosis, Evaluation, and Treatment of Attention-Deficit/Hyperactivity Disorder in Children and Adolescents', *Pediatrics* 128 (5): 1077–22. http://pediatrics.aappublications.org/content/128/5/1007.full.html (accessed 18 July 2013).

*Attention Deficit Hyperactivity Disorder: Diagnosis and Management of ADHD in Children, Young People and Adults.* Issued: September 2008; last modified: March 2013. NICE Clinical Guideline 72. www.guidance.nice.org.uk/cg72 (accessed 18 July 2013).

# Emotional regulation and behaviour

Difficulties of emotional regulation and behaviour are common and affect children's day-to-day function. For some children these difficulties may indicate the presence of a developmental disorder. A structured enquiry and observation are helpful in deciding about the level of reassurance, advice or the need for a referral for further assessment and management

**Typical developmental pattern – emotional regulation and behaviour**

- From birth to about 12 months parents help children manage their emotions by soothing or distracting them.

- From about 12 months onwards children begin to 'check-back' (*social referencing*) and begin to comply with caregivers' requests. Parents, sometimes, by ignoring children's emotional outbursts, give a message that a particular emotional response does not get attention.

- By 24 months children acquire some self-control over their behaviour by delaying action on request.

- As children improve in their language understanding parents help them manage their emotions by providing reassurance (e.g. 'I know you are sad but you are going to be alright'), alternative meaning of an emotional stimulus (e.g. '– did not mean to upset you') or other alternatives (e.g. 'why don't we make a card to say that you are sorry').

- From 3 years of age children show capability to modify behaviour based on situational rules (active play on the playground/ sitting and paying attention in class). They now seek help in stressful situations.

- Gradually, by the age of 4–5 years, the control of emotional expression shifts from needing external help to internalised self-regulation and based on understanding and reasoning (Thompson *et al.* 2013). They also begin to hide or modulate their emotions in a socially appropriate manner.

**Systematic enquiry**

Onset and duration of concerns regarding emotional difficulties are important to note as transient problems often arise due to change of social or physical circumstances, e.g. change of house, ill health or other changes in family dynamics. Concerns regarding behaviour usually start from the second year onwards. Information about behaviour in different settings, e.g. school or playgroup, social information such as family dynamics and how different family members respond to the problem, is useful in determining the type of problem and its functional impact.

Enquiry of carers starts with open-ended questions in order to elicit any concerns:

- Are you concerned about your child's behaviour? If so, what is the behaviour problem, how long has it gone on for, what seems to trigger the behaviour and how do you deal with it?

- Is your child aggressive, e.g. often fights with others, hurts others or seems spiteful towards others?

- Are you concerned that your child is unhappy, sad or tearful? If yes, for how long?

- Does your child often seem worried? If yes, in what situations?

- Are you concerned that your child is too fearful? If yes, in what situations?

- Has your child ever intentionally hurt himself (self-injury)?

**Observation (or enquiry of the carer)**

Children express frequent changes of feelings, mood, anxiety and fears in their facial expressions, gestures, voice and words, e.g. becoming excited about playing with a toy and sulking when they don't get what they want; hiding behind their parents before grad-ually settling to participate in activities. Interpreting an emotion is

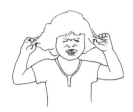

*anxious, fearful or angry? – interpretation of the same behaviour depends on context*

a somewhat subjective decision. Behaviour as observed should be noted first before describing the observer's and parent's interpretation. Any changes in behaviour are noted with change of activity, situations or with any parent–child interaction.

- What seemed to trigger the behaviour

- How did the caregiver respond?

- How long did the behaviour last?

- What helped in managing it?

- How did it affect the child's performance?

## Making observations of children's emotional regulation

Emotional expression and behaviour are observed during the examination of any developmental domain. However, these observations are often best made in natural settings of home, nursery/school or a playground. Validity and usefulness of the observations are improved by repeating observations over time and adhering to some basic principles such as:

- Observing both the behaviour and the context. Context is often the most important influence on a child's behaviour.

- Avoiding pre-existing expectations about certain behaviours from a child as this may affect the way you approach the child.

- Making objective observations and avoiding opinion and assumption, e.g. 'the child took the toy from the sibling' rather than 'the child behaved selfishly', 'the child was crying' rather than 'the child was sad', 'the child ran around the room for some/most of the time' rather than 'the child was hyperactive'. Interpretations of the behaviours observed may require a synthesis of information from multiple informants across different settings.

- The tasks offered to the child when his/her behaviour becomes negative must be developmentally appropriate.

- Mostly the reason for poor emotional regulation is the interaction between the child-related factors and the environmental stresses arising due to poor parenting or family dysfunction, poor socio-economic circumstances and task or situational demands.

- Most behaviour is open to change – by helping the child and parents and considering ways of reducing stresses. A multidisciplinary approach involving primary care health professionals, teachers and child and family services is often required to address significant concerns.

- Children with developmental disorders may have difficulty in generating alternative behaviours in response to admonishments and limits set by carers; such children may require specific intervention techniques, e.g. use of visual supports for children with autistic spectrum disorders.

- Change in the child's behaviour with the change in task demands or the type of activity, e.g. switching from verbal to non-verbal or play-based interactions may indicate underlying developmental difficulties. The child may simply be avoiding an experience of failure by refusing or creating diversions, e.g. becoming aggressive.

**Poor emotional regulation – management considerations**

Parental sensitivity and their responses to the child's behaviour are important indicators of parent–child interaction. Parental negativity towards the child, as expressed in their description of the child or as observed in their misattribution of the child's behaviour, e.g. believing that the child intentionally upsets them, may be a cause for concern. However, it should be remembered that the observations of parent–child interactions in structured or artificial settings may not necessarily be representative of those normally taking place at home (Gardner 2000) and a simplistic interpretation of the parent–child interaction can do more harm than good through misattribution of causal links or consequences.

**Observing parent-child interaction**

Observations can be made of the following:

Child

- seeking proximity following any stressful experience;
- showing affection towards parents;
- any negative behaviour towards parents, e.g. avoidance or withdrawal;
- persistent attempts to control the parents, e.g. by being punitive or solicitous;
- seeking undue proximity and affection from unfamiliar adults.

Parent

- how a parent approaches or responds to the child, e.g. greeting or physical proximity seeking (hugging, comforting);
- their emotional response, e.g. being happy/positive or frightened or uncertain;
- being consistent/inconsistent in their responses, e.g. praising and encouraging or mocking or teasing the child or pushing the child away;
- showing sudden mood changes or giving contradictory signals to the child – inviting and then rejecting the child or laughing at the child's distress;
- showing appropriate limit setting and rewards for the child's behaviour;
- showing any role confusion, e.g. pleading with the child, threatening to cry or talking as if the child is an adult partner.

Parental descriptions of the child also give clinically relevant information about the parent–child relationship. The key points which would raise concerns regarding the parent–child relationship are (Zenah *et al.* 2011):

- lack of positive description of the child;

- indifferent, hostile or impersonal description of the child;

- expression of shame, guilt or disappointment about the child;

- expressions of anger, hostility or disappointment about the child's needs, described as burdensome or overwhelming, or failure to imagine the child's needs;

- description of the child as a friend, peer or confidant;

- dissonance between a 'loving' description of their feelings for the child and indifferent or hostile description of the child.

# Physical examination and investigations

Physical examination is done by an appropriately qualified practitioner – e.g. GP, paediatrician, nurse practitioner, child psychiatrist or paediatric neurologist – primarily to look for a cause and/or for any other disorders associated with developmental impairments. The clinician undertaking the examination explains the purpose to parents. What has been done and its results are shared with parents and other clinicians, as relevant.

**Physical examination**

Physical examination has a limited but important role in the clinical evaluation of children with likely developmental problems (Majnemer and Shevell 1995). It can contribute to:

a. Providing cues for the cause of developmental impairment, e.g. dysmorphic features prompting a genetic test (Toriello 2008), small head circumference in foetal alcohol syndrome and, somewhat rarely, abnormal skin markings as an indicator for Tuberous Sclerosis.

b. Identifying any associated neurological impairment with the presenting developmental impairment, e.g. abnormal eye movements, large head, coarse features, liver enlargement or motor impairment in metabolic disorders; *hypotonia* in cerebellar problems and proximal muscle weakness in Duchenne muscular dystrophy.

c. Identifying the cause for a change of behaviour in children who are unable to communicate verbally, e.g. constipation, painful joint or tooth abscess.

d. Self-inflicted injuries may be observed in some children with developmental impairment, e.g. biting fingers, pulling out hair, poking eyes.

e. Providing information related to care or neglect (hygiene, growth) or features of physical abuse.

The most relevant aspects of physical examination of children presenting with developmental concerns are:

- Does the child look well cared for?

- Nutrition and growth – height and weight – to be plotted on WHO growth chart.

- Head circumference – to be plotted on WHO growth chart.

- Dysmorphic features (Table 8).

- *Gait* for ataxia.

- Observing the child picking something off the floor to exclude proximal weakness.

- Abnormal eye movements.

- Abnormal reflexes, tone, power, posture and movements.

- Any associated stereotypical motor movements, motor or vocal tics.

- Any evidence suggestive of non-accidental injury.

Neurological soft signs (e.g. dysdiadochokinesis, mirror movements) are commonly found in pre-school children with developmental difficulties but are non-specific for diagnostic purposes (Fellick *et al.* 2001).

## Planning investigations

Investigation planning, undertaken by a doctor, is a set of clinical decisions that are aided but not dictated by protocols (Palfrey and Frazer 2000; Moeschler 2008; Moeschler and Shevell, 2006). In the absence of an obvious cause, e.g. complications of pre-maturity, birth trauma or brain injury (although consider whether the cause is insufficient for the degree of delay), a constellation of features such as the course and severity of developmental difficulties, examination findings, knowledge of likely causes and associations and the impact of the investigation results on subsequent management influence the initial investigation plan. First-line genetic and other investigations (Box 4) followed by other tests, as indicated, in a stepwise manner is a sensible approach. Finding an underlying cause is most likely for severe cognitive impairment (global developmental delay) with an approximate yield of 50 per cent, particularly when associated with other findings from history and examination, e.g. dysmorphism or abnormal motor findings; while isolated language delays have a low diagnostic yield (Majnemer and Shevell, 1995).

*Table 8* Dysmorphic features – some examples of related syndromes.

| | | |
|---|---|---|
| **Hair** | Curly and coarse | Ectodermal dysplasias, Noonan syndrome |
| | Premature greying | Ataxia telangieactsia, Cockayne, Waardenburg syndrome |
| **Skull** | Microcephaly | FAS, CMV, herpes simplex and valproate, Aicardi-Goutieres, Angelman syndrome, skeletal dysplasia |
| | Macrocephaly | Achondroplasia, Noonan syndrome, NF1, Fragile X, Hypomelanosis of Ito |
| | Craniosynostosis | Apert's, Crouzon, Acrocephalosyndactyly, Smith-Magenis |
| **Ears** | Small | Associated with deafness, Treacher Collins, Facio-cardio-renal, Goldenhar syndrome |
| | Large | Fragile X; association with multiple congenital anomalies, learning disability and cerebral palsy |
| | Low set | Multiple syndromes associated with deafness and/or other systemic abnormalities, e.g. CHARGE association, FG syndrome |
| | Preauricular pits and tags | Syndromes associated with deafness, seizures, learning disability, cardiac defects and other systemic anomalies, Brachio-oto-renal syndrome |
| **Eyebrows** | Joined | Cornelia de Lange, Waardenburg |
| **Eyes** | Prominent eyes | Craniosynostosis, Apert's, Crouzon |
| | Upslanting eyes | DS, Trisomy 9 |
| | Downslanting eyes | Noonan, Marfan's, craniosynostosis |
| | Epicanthic folds | FAS, DS |
| **Nose** | Flat nasal bridge | DS |
| | Short nose | FAS, William's syndrome |

| | Anteverted nares | Cornelia de Lange |
| | Short and smooth philtrum | FAS |
| **Face** | Frontal bossing | Sotos syndrome |
| | Flat malar bones | DS, Treacher Collins syndrome |
| | Prominent cheekbones | William's syndrome |
| **Mouth** | Thin upper lips | FAS |
| | Bow-shaped lips | Smith-Magenis syndrome |
| **Neck** | Webbed neck and low posterior hairline | Noonan, Turner |
| **Limbs** | Asymmetric lower limbs | Hemihyperplasia, Russell Silver syndrome, Hypomelanosis of Ito |
| **Hands** | Small hands and feet | Prader-Willi syndrome, metaphyseal dysplasia |
| | Unusual palmar creases | DS, FAS, Cranioectodermal dysplasia |
| **Nails** | Hypoplasia | FAS, foetal cocaine effects, cutis/skeletal dysplasia |
| | Periungual fibroma | Tuberous sclerosis |
| **Skin** | Hypopigmented (ash leaf) macules, adenoma sebaceum on malar region | Tuberous sclerosis |
| | Cafe au lait marks >1.5 cm and freckling in the armpits | NF1 |
| | Port wine stain (overlying part of the ophthalmic branch of the trigeminal nerve on the face) | Sturge Weber syndrome |
| | Photosensitivity | Chromosome breakage disorders |
| **Genitalia** | Small | Prader-Willi syndrome, adrenal hypoplasia |
| | Large testicles | Fragile X syndrome |

CMV: cytomegalovirus, DS: Down's syndrome, FAS: foetal alcohol syndrome, NF1: Neurofibromatosis 1.

---

**BOX 4** Investigations for moderate to severe global cognitive impairment[1] (functioning at approximately < 70 per cent of chronological age in two or more domains)

- Array CGH or chromosome analysis where a CGH not available
- Fragile X[2]
- CK in boys
- Thyroid function test

Additional investigations for specific indications:

a. Infants, under 2 years of age, with microcephaly and intrauterine growth retardation (IUGR):

- Toxoplasma and rubella assay and urine CMV culture

b. Dysmorphic features: referral/consultation with a geneticist

c. Behaviour suggestive of seizures, behavioural phenotype of Angelman syndrome:

- Electroencephalogram (EEG)

d. Neurological deterioration, focal neurological features:

- Referral to neurologist
- Neuroimaging

e. Features suggestive of metabolic cause, e.g. failure to thrive, organomegaly, coarse features, history suggestive of metabolic decompensation, family history of consanguinity, neonatal deaths, life-threatening episodes in siblings:

- Amino acids, urine organic acids, mucopolysaccharides, urates, biotinidase, urine purine (consider the most appropriate investigations in consultation with a paediatric metabolic specialist)

f. Consider if any concern regarding general health, diet or growth:

- FBC, serum ferritin, vitamin D

[1] Investigations for lesser degrees of developmental impairment are guided by associated clinical findings, e.g. dysmorphism, neurological or other systemic or psychological features.

[2] Fragile X: most likely in children with two or more of the following features: moderate to severe developmental delay, features of autistic spectrum disorder (ASD), social anxiety, long ears (after 7 years), large testicles (post-pubertal), family history of learning difficulties. It is unlikely to be present in children with classic aloof autism or Asperger's syndrome.

http://ukgtn.nhs.uk/find-a-test/search-by-disorder-gene/#c3662 (information regarding genetic testing).

Analysis and management | **Section 3**

# Making sense of findings

Previous chapters have outlined different aspects of clinical evaluation of children's development. In summary, these have encompassed:

- eliciting concerns from parents/carers;

- noting medical or psycho-social risk factors;

- information regarding the child's current functioning (academic, social-behavioural or daily life activities) and any informal observation of the child;

- structured observation of developmental abilities;

- physical examination;

- investigations.

The next task for a practitioner is to synthesise the available information and make decisions regarding some key questions about a child's developmental function:

- Is there an impairment of a child's expected developmental function in one or more domains? If so:

  - Is the degree of variation significant?

  - Is there any qualitative impairment of function?

  - Is there a likelihood of an underlying or associated neuro-developmental disorder?

- Are there significant *functional difficulties* in learning, communicating, socialising or activities of daily living?

- Are there any adverse social circumstances likely to be affecting development?

- Does the presenting profile of development create any long-term *vulnerability* for the child? For example, children with impaired language or fine motor skills are more likely to develop attention, reading, behaviour and social problems (Snowling *et al.* 2006; Cantell and Kooistra 2002). This probabilistic understanding should be shared with parents, without raising undue anxieties, and anticipatory help and guidance provided for improving the child's outcomes.

- Are any further specialists assessments required?

- Would the child benefit from any additional support or intervention? If so, do the parents agree to further referrals and sharing of information?

- What further information and support can be provided to parents?

**Clinical decision-making – assessing the significance of findings**

The task of deciding when a child's developmental progress is significantly impaired is made difficult by the wide normal variation in the typical development. Any simplistic approach of using numbers to describe the ratio or proportion of developmental variation has a risk of giving an undue air of objectivity and ignoring other aspects of findings, e.g. poor function in the real-life settings. Also, it should be recognised that children may simply not perform well during observations due to an unfamiliar setting or other anxieties (either their own, or their parents'/carers'). It is the nature of development, with all its variations, that makes the interpretation of findings probabilistic, no matter how standardised the test.

Clinical interpretation is based on an understanding of children's developmental progress and knowledge regarding variations, functional difficulties and profiles of neuro-developmental examination indicative of developmental vulnerabilities and disorders, some examples of which are the following:

1. The degree of variation

The significance of a delay in achieving *developmental milestones* depends on the age of the child; for example, a three month delay is more significant during infancy than during the second year or later. Also, the presence or absence of other risk factors would influence whether a delay is likely to persist. While a severe delay (e.g. a child functioning at a developmental level less than half their age or crossing 'red flag' ages for key milestones in one or more domains) is mostly predictive of persisting difficulties, lesser degrees of delay can often be transient. However, children with lesser degrees of variation may also be in need of help if associated with social or biological risk factors and/or associated with *functional difficulties*.

The term 'developmental delay' is not always helpful. Any variation or delay in development is a symptom, not a diagnosis, and it may be transient or long-lasting. The implication of the word 'delay' is that the thing that is delayed will eventually arrive, and the child will catch up with his/her peers. For children with persisting developmental disorders this may be a false expectation. The majority of children, in the absence of *neurodegenerative* conditions, will continue to make progress, although perhaps at a slower rate than their peers, resulting in an increasing gap between the achievements of an individual child and those expected in the typical population. The focus may be better placed on identifying any impairment of the expected function and its qualitative aspects, while it may be appropriate to refer to any delay in a specific domain of development as contributing to the impairment.

2. Qualitative variations

Some children present with differences in not just what they can do but how they do it. Such qualitative differences may indicate the likelihood of a neurodevelopmental disorder, particularly if they cause functional difficulties. Common examples of such qualitative observations are:

a. a lack of social awareness and poor quality of interactions, particularly with peers;
b. taking excessive interest in a narrow range of objects or activities;
c. a high level of *impulsivity* or poor attention to tasks;
d. unusual sensory interests or aversions (e.g. extreme food faddiness, hypersensitivity to sounds, avoidance of touch, etc.);
e. poor planning or organising.

3. Neuro-developmental profiles suggestive of disorders/vulnerabilities

A pattern of impairment or delay, combined with findings from inquiry and examination, can be a helpful guide for identifying likely causes and in making decisions regarding further assessment/investigations (Tervo 2006).

**A. Global developmental impairment**

Defined as a significant delay in two or more of the major developmental domains (gross/fine motor, speech/language, cognitive, social, and self-care or activities of daily living), although most affected children have significant impairment evident in all five of the domains.

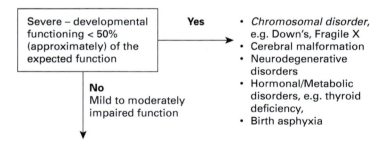

## B. Mainly single-domain impairments

### 1. Language impairment

Language is a cognitive function, therefore any cognitive impairment (learning disability) will impact on language learning. In order to diagnose speech and language disorders consideration must be given to the child's level of cognitive ability (verbal and non-verbal). The following decision tree suggests the most likely queries, arising from the presenting pattern of impairments requiring appropriate further assessment (Bishop 2002).

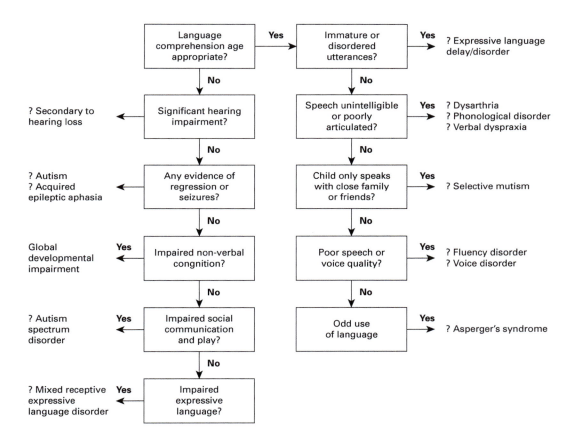

2. Impaired gross motor function

The causes of impaired motor function presenting as delayed motor development range from benign familial patterns, e.g. bottom-shuffling, to severe neurological and/or systemic disorders. Careful general and systemic examination is required to guide the clinician towards the most likely cause (Table 9).

3. Impaired fine motor function – likely causes or associated conditions

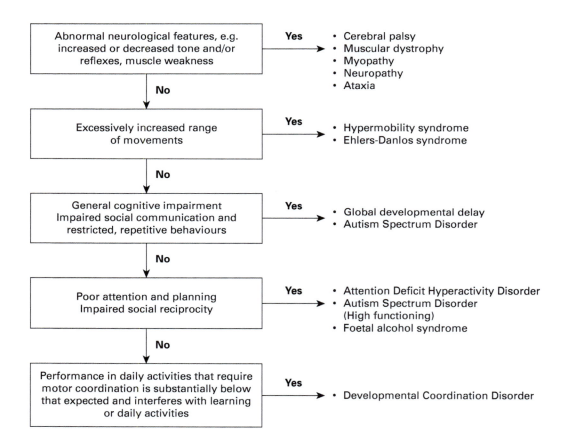

Table 9 Leading causes of motor impairment based on clinical features.

| Impaired cognition | Dysmorphic features | Abnormal tone and/or reflexes | Muscle weakness | Family history | Other | |
|---|---|---|---|---|---|---|
| + | | | | | | GDD (see above for causes) |
| + | + | + Hypotonia | | | | Down's, P-W and William's syndromes |
| +/- | | + ↑ or variable tone | | | +/- seizures | Cerebral palsy, brain malformation |
| | | + Hypotonia | + | | | Congenital muscular dystrophies (e.g. Duchenne) |
| | | + Hypotonia Areflexia | + | | Muscle fasciculations | Spinal muscular atrophy |
| | | + | + | + | | Congenital myotonia, myopathies |
| | | + Hypotonia | | +/- ↑ if consanguineous parents | Abn. liver function; +/- seizures | Metabolic, myesthenia |
| | | + | + (in legs) | | Abn. spine, bladder, bowel and feet | Spina bifida occulta |
| | | | | | Poor vision | Visual impairment |
| | | | | + | | Familial; bottom shuffling |

Abn.: abnormal; GDD: global developmental delay; P-W: Prader-Willi syndrome.

## C. Plateauing or regression

Transient lack of participation or withdrawal from activities, such as communication (e.g. transient selective mutism), is often seen following any significant social-emotional upheaval in a child's life. Regression is considered to be present when there is a loss of previously acquired developmental skills following a period of normal or delayed development. The following patterns of presentations are seen in regression:

1. Most commonly, a loss of language, communication and social skills is seen between 15 to 24 months in 20–30 per cent of children presenting with autism spectrum disorders (ASD).

The following presentations are rare, but are important to consider for their early identification:

2. Children with Landau Kleffener Syndrome (LKS) or acquired epileptic aphasia present with language regression between the age of 2 and 8 years (peak age is 4–5 years), accompanied by epileptiform EEG abnormalities and/ or clinical seizures (in 70–80 per cent). The language disturbance is severe receptive language deficit or 'word deafness'. They do not lose reciprocal social interaction skills and do not have repetitive or restricted interests or behaviours, in contrast to ASD with regression.

3. Electrical Status Epilepticus in Sleep (ESES) or continuous spike wave during slow wave sleep (CSWS) is an epileptic disorder, presenting in the age group 1–14 years (mean 4–8 years, characterised by specific EEG abnormalities. It is associated with language (expressive aphasia), cognitive (decline in non-verbal abilities) and behavioural features (e.g. inattention, disinhibition, aggression) and motor abnormalities (e.g. ataxia, dystonia, dyspraxia).

4. Childhood Disintegrative Disorder: presents after apparently normal development up to the age of at least 2 years and is followed by a significant loss, over a few months, in at least several areas of development: language, play, social skills,

adaptive behaviour, bowel or bladder control, and sometimes, motor skills.

5. Progressive regression is often indicative of a degenerative neurological cause and requires an urgent referral to a paediatric neurologist.

**D. Functional difficulties** in communication, movement, coordination or learning in real-life settings, e.g. school, and any risk-taking behaviour need referral for specialist assessments (e.g. speech and language therapy, occupational therapy, physiotherapy) even where there is no specific diagnosis or significant delay.

**Caveats and limitations**

Development is rapidly changing over time for a given child, with large variations within the population and for the same child. A single developmental examination only gives a view of the child's abilities at that time. The long-term stability of a one-off developmental score is limited (Darrah *et al.* 2003). This limits the sensitivity and specificity of any developmental examination measure or method and, at least initially, the interpretation is often presumptive. At least some acknowledgement of this should be made in discussion with parents and in reports. Some other specific limitations to consider are:

- ■ *Narrow focus:* Identification of developmental delay may not be the most useful activity, as the delay in some cases may be a short-term phenomenon, while in other cases qualitative developmental impairment may be present without any 'delay'. A narrow focus on the child's difficulties in one particular domain, without attention to other factors, may also lead to a wrong conclusion such as diagnosing developmental delay in the presence of sensory impairment or poor social environment.

- ■ *Setting:* Clinical settings are different from natural environments in which young children typically function and may affect their performance significantly.

- ■ Children's performance may be affected by other factors, e.g. anxiety or poor attention.

## Consideration of child abuse and neglect

Child maltreatment has short- and long-term medical, mental health, and social sequelae (Dubowitz and Bennett 2007). Abused or neglected children are at risk of developing health-related, developmental, behavioural and functional difficulties, including conduct disorders, aggressive behaviours, decreased cognitive functioning, inappropriate sexual behaviour and poor academic achievement. All practitioners working with children have a role in preventing abuse and neglect by supporting families at the earliest opportunity. All have a responsibility for early identification and timely intervention where abuse or neglect may be present.

*Practice issues*

The key issue is the preparedness of practitioners to contemplate the possibility that a child's presentation could, at least in part, be explained by abuse or neglect (Gilbert *et al.* 2009). They should have the required knowledge and skills, an awareness of the local child protection policy and procedures and have access to consultation with their seniors and/or the local child protection team.

Early identification of abuse or neglect is helped by:

■ an appraisal of existing information about the child and the family, e.g. if they were previously known to services with presentations which may be due to neglect or abuse;

■ consideration of chid-related vulnerability factors, e.g.:

- ■ disability or special educational needs (NSPCC 2007)

- ■ risk-taking or antisocial behaviour

- ■ being a young carer

- ■ presenting with an injury for which there is no explanation, or changing explanations, or with an injury that is inconsistent with the child's developmental abilities (e.g. injuries in infants who are not independently mobile), and/or the type or distribution of the injury

■ consideration of carer/family-related vulnerability factors, e.g.:

- family circumstance presenting challenges for the child, such as substance abuse, adult mental health problems, domestic violence, parent or carer with a learning disability, history of poor parenting or previous involvement with child protection services;

- inappropriate parent or carer response (unconcerned or aggressive) to presenting concerns.

Where practitioners have any concerns about child abuse or neglect they should have a low threshold for consulting with their seniors and/or the specialist child protection team at the earliest opportunity.

**Factors that reduce the effectiveness of developmental examination**

- Lack of collaborative working and/or sharing of information with other professionals

- Difficulty in distinguishing fact from opinion

- Working from assumptions rather than evidence

- Inadequate knowledge of patterns of developmental progress

- Difficulty in interpreting, or understanding, the information that is available

- Difficulty in identifying what is significant

- Over-confidence in the certainty of an assessment.

**Referral pathways**

Deciding where to refer a child is a matter of professional judgement, parental agreement and knowledge of local services and referral pathways. Some key considerations in making this decision are:

- Paying attention to parental concerns, particularly regarding hearing and vision to refer for an audiological/orthoptic assessment.

- Consider making referral for both a general (e.g. community paediatrician) and a specific (speech and language therapist, mental health services etc.) assessment if the concern is in more than one domain.

- Explaining to parents/carers why the referral is being made and what is expected from a particular service.

- Providing parents with information and contacts of the services to which the child is being referred.

- Providing parents with support and guidance for helping the child's development and behaviour.

**Further reading**

Aicardi, J. (2009) *Diseases of the Nervous System in Childhood*, 3rd edn. London: MacKeith Press.

*Child Protection Companion* (2013) London: Royal College of Paediatrics and Child Health.

Glaser, D. (2008) 'Child Maltreatment', *Psychiatry* 7 (7): 295–8.

Seal, A., Robinson, G., Kelly, A. M. and Williams, J. (2013) *Children with Neurodevelopmental Disabilities: The Essential Guide to Assessment and Management*. London: MacKeith Press.

*When to Suspect Child Maltreatment, NICE Guidance G89* (2009). London: National Collaborating Centre for Women's and Children's Health. http://www.nice.org.uk/nicemedia/live/12183/44914/44914.pdf (accessed 30 July 2013).

Woolraich, M. L., Drotar, D. D., Dworkin, P. H. and Perrin, E. C. (2008) *Developmental Behavioural Pediatrics: Evidence and Practice*. Philadelphia, PA: Mosby Elsevier.

# Communicating with parents/carers

It is important for the child that professionals and parents/carers work together when addressing any developmental or behavioural concerns. Yet it can sometimes be difficult to make an enquiry of parents, share with them any areas of concern about their child or suggest ways of helping the child (see Barriers to parents raising concerns or accessing services, p. 6) (Glascoe and Marks 2011).

Parents react in different ways: some parents may feel blamed or angry while others may feel relief and be grateful for the chance to share concerns and seek support for their child. Studies exploring the value of early screening for children with developmental disorders have raised questions about whether it is appropriate or helpful to alert parents to problems before they themselves have suspicions that all is not well (Baird *et al.* 2001). However, talking with parents about their child is an opportunity for professionals to establish a partnership that works for improving the outcome for the child, which is crucial for their engagement with services. The following general principles are helpful in achieving this:

- Good communication skills, establishing trust and openness to negotiating are the basic principles for working with parents. Acknowledging the language barrier and using interpreters is essential for good communication.

- Listening to parents and encouraging them to talk sets up a good starting point. Finding out what is known and what is wanted – how ready the parents are – enables the practitioner to negotiate a constructive approach. Parents may be anxious, embarrassed or sad and the practitioner needs to understand their viewpoint and priorities.

- Keep the focus of any discussion on helping the child.

- Summarise the information you have gathered – refer to records to check accuracy. Use clear and simple language – explaining any medical term.

- Give information in small chunks. Repeat any important points. Pause often to allow questions.

- Acknowledge the limits of the enquiry/examination and recognise room for errors.

- Act professionally: if you cannot answer a question do not waffle or evade; suggest that you would take note and come back to them.

- It may be helpful to discuss findings with a more experienced colleague before making an onward referral. A second session with another colleague (either a more senior colleague or one from a different profession) may be indicated if there are gaps in the information gleaned from the initial contact.

- Don't argue with parents when they tell you that you are wrong; encourage them to talk to another professional. Be thoughtful and caring in your approach. Be prepared for a range of responses from parents, e.g. anger, blame or denial.

- Be positive: value the child; identify and reinforce parental strengths; identify other sources of support – parent to parent, voluntary, services.

- Be honest without being unkind.

- Reinforce with written information (providing translations where required).

- Finish communication in a positive way with a plan. Offer to discuss again and arrange another meeting if needed.

**Resources**

*Right from the Start Template – Good Practice in Sharing the News* (2003) London: Scope. http://www.scope.org.uk/sites/default/files/pdfs/Early _years/Scope_Right_from_the_Start_template.pdf (accessed 30 July 2013).

Resources | **Section 4**

# Internet resources

http://www.afasicengland.org.uk/

Afasic is a UK charity which supports children and young people with speech, language and communication impairments and their parents and carers. Information on language development and disorders and how to get help.

http://www.ican.org.uk/

I CAN is a UK charity aiming to support the development of all children's speech, language and communication, focusing particularly on those with communication disorders. Provider of information and direct services. Resources include free DVDs:

- *Chatter Matters*: advice for parents on supporting language development.

- *Learning to Talk*: for early years professionals.

www.education.gov.uk/publications/standard/publicationDetail/Page1/DEVELOPMENT-MATTERS

The Early Years Foundation Stage (EYFS) is the statutory framework that sets the standards that all Early Years providers must meet to ensure that children learn and develop well and are kept healthy and safe. Development Matters in the Early Years Foundation Stage provides guidance to support practitioners in implementing those statutory requirements.

http://developingchild.harvard.edu/

A great source of up-to-date scientific information about child development with multimedia resources.

http://www.literacytrust.org.uk/talk_to_your_baby

A campaign run by the National Literacy Trust to encourage parents and carers to talk more to children from birth to 3 years. Useful information sheets on early communication and on development of reading and writing. Also resources on attachment.

www.socialbaby.com

The website of The Children's Project. A source of books and materials for parents with young children, and professionals supporting and promoting early years development. Resources include books and DVDs:

- *Baby and Me* – in English; Arabic and Sylheti; Polish and Portuguese
- *The Social Toddler*

www.tt4tt.co.uk

Website of The Learning Partnership, a social interest company. The Top Tips for Tiny Tots site offers a 'course' via animations on strategies that parents can use to encourage development of intelligence.

www.talkingpoint.org.uk

Joint website developed by ICAN, Afasic and the Royal College of Speech and Language Therapists, giving information on language development, recognition and support for those with language difficulties. Sections for parents, early years workers, therapists, GPs, teachers. Resources include online games and picture materials designed to support early language skills.

http://www.canchild.ca/en/

The Canchild website from McMasters University has good resources regarding Developmental Coordination Disorder, from research to general advice, etc.

www.infantandtoddlerforum.org

Advice on nutrition in young children, including managing common feeding difficulties in toddlers.

http://www.nlm.nih.gov/medlineplus/childdevelopment.html#cat1 and www.cdc.gov/ncbddd/child

US websites for information on overview, initiatives and information regarding child development.

http://www.cafamily.org.uk/

Information and resources for children with disabilities and special needs

http://www.education.gov.uk/aboutdfe/statutory/g00213160/ working-together-to-safeguard-children

HM Government, *Working Together to Safeguard Children* (March 2013). Stationery Office, London, UK.

http://www.nice.org.uk/nicemedia/live/12183/44914/44914.pdf

*When to Suspect Child Maltreatment*, NICE Guidance G89 (2009). National Collaborating Centre for Women's and Children's Health, UK.

http://www.aussiechildcarenetwork.com/child_stages_of_ development.php

Australian website of resources and information regarding child development.

# Glossary

The words from this Glossary can be found either in the text, the companion website and/or the accompanying videos.

**Agency:** the idea that people make events happen through their internal motivation.

**Apgar scale:** a rating system used to assess a newborn baby's physical condition immediately after birth on the basis of five characteristics: heart rate, respiratory effort, reflex irritability, muscle tone and colour.

**Attention:** concentration and focusing of mental resources.

**Audiometry:** the testing of a person's ability to hear various sound frequencies. The test is performed an audiometer.

**Babble:** infant's vocalisation of reduplicated sequences of consonant–vowel syllables which function as the building blocks of words.

**Cephalocaudal pattern:** muscle tone and strength develop first in the muscles supporting the head and gradually spread towards feet.

**Chromosomal disorders:** a chromosome abnormality reflects an abnormality of chromosome number (missing a chromosome, e.g. Turner syndrome, or having an extra chromosome, e.g. Down's syndrome) or structure (e.g. deletion, duplication or translocation of part of a chromosome).

**Cognition:** psychological processes that lead to 'knowing', e.g. attending, remembering, symbolising.

**Concept vocabulary:** words indicating the location of objects (as opposed to object names), e.g. high, low, top, down, under.

**Contexts:** unique combinations of personal and environmental circumstances that can result in different paths of development, e.g. historical, family, economic and social factors.

**Cooperative play:** play that involves social interaction in a group, with a sense of organised activity.

**Definition-by-use:** child, when given an object, plays with it in an appropriate way, e.g. spoon in the mouth, brush on hair.

**Developmental milestones:** a developmental ability that is achieved by most children at a certain age.

**Domain-specific:** related to a specific domain of development, e.g. language or fine motor.

**Dynamic:** continuous and systemic process of change and development.

**Echoing:** repeating what someone says.

**Epigenetic effects:** epigenetic effects are variations which are transmitted from parent to offspring but are not caused by DNA nucleotide sequence changes (substitutions, losses, etc.). They are rather due to environmental effects on gene function or expression.

**Executive functions:** the monitoring and self-regulation of thought and action, to plan behaviour and to inhibit inappropriate response.

**Facilitative guidance:** general guidance to parents and carers to promote the child's development.

**False belief:** an understanding that others may have beliefs that do not reflect current reality.

**Functional difficulties:** reported difficulties in day-to-day activities, e.g. playing, communicating, learning or socialising.

**Gait:** a person's manner of walking.

**Genetic expression:** the process by which information from a gene is used in the synthesis of a functional gene product, e.g. proteins, hormones and enzymes.

**Gestational age:** the duration of pregnancy (and thus the age of a foetus), measured from the 'first day of the last normal menstrual period'.

**Global developmental delay:** impairment of developmental progress in two or more domains (involving aspects of both verbal and non-verbal development).

**Guttural sounds:** sounds produced at the back of the mouth, usually vowels and usually of a harsh quality.

**Hypothalamic Pituitary Adrenal (HPA) axis:** the HPA axis refers to the hypothalamic-pituitary-adrenocortical axis. It is the internal neuroendocrine system that responds to stress and results in production of corticosteroid hormones that affect the brain, the cardiovascular system, and other systems in getting the body ready for what is known as the 'fight or flight' mechanism.

**Hypo/hypertonia:** decreased/increased muscle tone.

**Impulsivity:** acting before thinking; erratic and poorly controlled behaviour.

**Intrinsic reinforcements:** inner satisfaction and enjoyment from completing a task as opposed to external rewards.

**Jargon:** 'conversational babbling' or pre-linguistic vocalisations of young children that consist of several strings of consonants and vowels and may sound like connected speech, even though they are not true words. Jargon may have stress and the intonation patterns of connected speech.

**Joint attention:** is the shared focus of two individuals on an object. It is achieved when one individual alerts another to an object by means of eye-gazing, pointing or other verbal or non-verbal indications.

**Make-believe play:** a type of play in which children act out everyday and imaginary activities.

**Metacognition:** being aware of one's own thought processes including identifying problems, formulating solutions to problems, and so forth.

**Micro/macrocephaly:** a head circumference (HC) more than 2 standard deviation below/above the mean for age and gender.

**Muscle tone:** the continuous and passive partial contraction of the muscles, or the muscles' resistance to passive stretch during resting state.

**Neonate:** infant within age range of birth to 4 weeks.

**Neurodegenerative disease:** diseases resulting in the progressive loss of structure or function of neurons.

**Neurotransmitters:** chemicals released by neurons that cross the synapse to send messages to other neurons.

**Norms/normative:** when and how most children achieve a developmental ability.

**Nystagmus:** rapid involuntary movements of the eyes.

**Object manipulation:** hand-guided motor actions such as coordinated looking, rotating, transferring and fingering that facilitate infants' understanding of objects and events involving objects.

**Operant conditioning:** a method of learning that occurs through rewards and punishments for behaviour. Through these rewards and punishments, an association is made between behaviour and a consequence for that behaviour.

**Perceptual feedback:** perception is influenced by expectation or belief; feedback from experience confirms or modifies such expectations or beliefs.

**Perinatal period:** the time period starting at 22 completed weeks' gestation and lasting through seven days after birth.

**Permanence of object/Object permanence:** the understanding that objects continue to exist when they are out of sight.

**Plasticity:** the potential for relative systematic change in human development across the lifespan.

**Popliteal angle:** the angle between thigh and calf (femur and tibia) measured in supine position with the hip flexed 90° and the knee extended.

**Premature (preterm):** infant born before 37 weeks of gestation.

**Pretend play:** play involving acting out ideas and emotions. Children act out actions and stories that contain different perspectives and ideas.

**Proprioception:** the ability to sense the position, location, orientation and movement of the body and its parts.

**Red flag:** a range of functional indicators or domains commonly used to monitor healthy child development, as well as potential problem areas for child development. It is intended to assist in the determination of when and where to refer for additional advice, formal assessment and/or treatment.

**Red reflex:** refers to the reddish-orange reflection of light from the eye's retina that is observed when using an ophthalmoscope from approximately 30 cm/1 foot.

**Scaffolding** is a process by which adults support and guide children's learning, enabling children to reach to the next level of ability, beyond their own personal capability at that time. The term was coined by Bruner, building on Vygotsky's work.

**Sensitive period:** a time that is optimal for certain developmental capacities to emerge and in which the individual is especially responsive to environmental influences.

**Sensitive-responsive parenting:** parents give positive affection and high levels of warmth to the child, respond sensitively and positively to the child's signals and acknowledge the child's unique identity. Sensitive-responsive parents maintain children's focus of interest and enhance their experience by providing rich verbal input in response.

**Social referencing:** using feedback from others to determine how to respond.

**Social smile:** the smile evoked by the stimulus of the human face. First appears between 6 and 10 weeks.

**Squint:** a deviation in the direction of the gaze of one eye.

**Stranger wariness:** expression of fear in response to unfamiliar adults, which appears in many babies in the second half of the first year.

**Theory of mind:** the ability to accredit mental states to self and others.

**Transactional process:** a mutually interactive process in which children and the environment simultaneously influence each other, producing developmental change in both over time.

**Visual acuity:** sharpness of vision, which may be measured by the ability to discern letters or numbers at a given distance according to a fixed standard.

**Vulnerability:** susceptible to poor developmental outcomes due to genetic, physical, cognitive or temperamental factors.

**Walking base:** describes how close (narrow base) or far apart (wide base) both legs are kept while walking.

**Working memory:** the memory system that temporarily keeps in information just received.

# References

Amiel-Tison, C. and Grenier, A. (1986) *Neurological Assessment during the First Year of Life*. New York: Oxford University Press.

Bada, H. S., Bann, C. M., Whitaker, T. M., Bauer, C. R., Shankaran, S., Lagasse, L., Lester, B. M., Hammond, J. and Higgins, R. (2012) 'Protective Factors Can Mitigate Behavior Problems after Prenatal Cocaine and Other Drug Exposures', *Pediatrics* 130 (6): e1479–88.

Baird, G., Charman, T., Baron-Cohen, S., Cox, A., Swettenham, J., Wheelwright, S. and Drew, A. (2001) 'Screening and Surveillance for Autism and Pervasive Developmental Disorders', *Archives of Disease in Childhood* 84: 468–75.

Bandura, A. (1989) 'Social Cognitive Theory', *Annals of Child Development* 6: 1–60.

Barth, R. P., Scarborough, A., Lloyd, E. C., Losby, J., Casanueva, C. and Mann, T. (2007) *Developmental Status and Early Intervention Service Needs of Maltreated Children*. Washington, DC: US Department of Health and Human Services, Office of the Assistant Secretary for Planning and Evaluation. http://aspe.hhs.gov/hsp/08/devneeds/report.pdf (accessed 30 July 2013).

Bishop, D. V. M. (2002) 'Speech and Language Difficulties', in M. Rutter and E. Taylor (eds), *Child and Adolescent Psychiatry: Modern Approaches*. Oxford: Blackwell, pp. 664–81.

Boyce, W. T. and Ellis, B. J. (2005) 'Biological Sensitivity to Context: I. An Evolutionary-Developmental Theory of the Origins and Functions of Stress Reactivity', *Development and Psychopathology* 17 (2): 271–301.

Bronfenbrenner, U. and Morris, P. A. (2006) 'The Bioecological Model of Human Development', in W. Damon and R. M. Lerner (eds), *Handbook of Child Psychology, Vol. 1: Theoretical Models of Human Development*, 6th edn. New York: John Wiley, pp. 793–828.

Cantell, M. and Kooistra, L. (2002) 'Long Term Outcomes of Developmental Coordination Disorder', in S. A. Cermak and D. Larkin (eds), *Developmental Coordination Disorder*. Albany, NY: Delmar Thomson Learning.

Capute, A. J. and Accardo, P. J. (1996) 'A Neurodevelopmental Perspective on the Continuum of Developmental Disabilities', in A. J. Capute and P. J. Accardo (eds), *Developmental Disabilities in Infancy and Childhood*, 2nd edn. Baltimore, MD: Paul H. Brookes, pp. 1–22.

Clarke, J. (2005) 'Locomotion', in B. Hopkins (ed.), *The Cambridge Encyclopaedia of Child Development*. Cambridge: Cambridge University Press, pp. 336–9.

Cole, M. and Packer, M. (2011) 'Culture in Development', in M. H. Bornstein and M. E. Lamb. *Cognitive Development and Advanced Textbook*. New York: Psychology Press, pp. 67–123.

Couperus, J. W. and Nelson, C. A. (2006) 'Early Brain Development and Plasticity', in K. McCartney and D. Phillips (eds), *The Blackwell Handbook of Early Childhood Development*. Oxford: Blackwell Press.

Daniel, B., Gilligan, R. and Wassel, S. (2010) *Child Development for Child Care and Protection Workers*, 2nd edn. London: Jessica Kingsley Publishers.

Darrah, J., Hodge, M., Magill-Evans, J. and Kembhavi, G. (2003) 'Stability of Serial Assessments of Motor and Communication Abilities in Typically Developing Infants – Implications for Screening', *Early Human Development* 72: 569–70.

Dooley, J. M., Gordon, K. E., Wood, E. P., Camfield, C. S. and Camfield, P. R. (2003) 'The Utility of the Physical Examination and Investigations in the Pediatric Neurology Consultation', *Pediatric Neurology* 28: 96–9.

Dubowitz, H. and Bennett, S. (2007) 'Physical Abuse and Neglect of Children', *The Lancet* 369 (9576): 1891–9.

Elder, G. H., Van Nguyen, T. and Caspi, A. (1985) 'Linking Family Hardships to Children's Lives', *Child Development* 56 (2): 361–75.

Evans, G. W. (2006) 'Child Development and the Physical Environment', *Annual Review of Psychology* 57: 423–51.

Fellick, J., Thomson, A., Sills, J. and Hart, C. A. (2001) 'Neurological Soft Signs in Mainstream Pupils', *Archives of Disease in Childhood* 85: 371–4.

Gardner, F. (2000) 'Methodological Issues in the Direct Parent–Child Interaction: Do Observational Findings Reflect the Natural Behaviour of Participants?', *Clinical Child and Family Psychology Review* 3: 185–98.

Garner, A. S., Shonkoff, J. P., Siegel, B. S., Dobbins, M. I., Earls, M. F., McGuinn, L., Pascoe, J. and Wood, D. L. (2012) 'Early Childhood Adversity, Toxic Stress, and the Role of the Pediatrician: Translating Developmental Science into Lifelong HEALTH', *Pediatrics* 129: e224.

Gilbert, R., Kemp, A., Thoburn, J., Sidebotham, P., Radford, L., Glaser, D. and MacMillan, H. L. (2009) 'Recognising and Responding to Child Maltreatment', *The Lancet* 373 (9658): 167–80.

Glascoe, F. P. (1994) 'It's Not What It Seems: The Relationship between Parents' Concerns and Children with Global Delays', *Clinical Pediatrics* 33: 292–6.

Glascoe, F. P. (1999) 'A Method for Deciding How to Respond to Parents' Concerns about Development and Behavior', *Ambulatory Child Health* 5: 197–208.

Glascoe, F. P. (2003) 'Parents' Evaluation of Developmental Status: How Well Do Parents' Concerns Identify Children with Behavioural and Emotional Problems?', *Clinical Pediatrics* 42: 133–8.

Glascoe, F. P. and Dworkin, P. (1993) 'Obstacles in Effective Developmental Surveillance: Errors in Clinical Reasoning', *Journal of Developmental and Behavioural Pediatrics* 14: 344–9.

Glascoe, F. P. and Leew, S. (2010) 'Parenting Behaviors, Perceptions, and Psychosocial Risk: Impacts on Young Children's Development', *Pediatrics* 125: 313–19.

Glascoe, F. P. and Marks, K. P. (2011) 'Detecting Children with Developmental Behavioral Problems: The Value of Collaborating with Parents', *Psychological Test and Assessment Modeling* 53 (2): 258–79.

Glascoe, F. P. and Sandler, H. (1995) 'Value of Parents' Estimates of Children's Developmental Ages', *Journal of Pediatrics* 127: 831–5.

Greenspan, S. and Meisels, S. (1996) 'Toward a New Vision for the Developmental Assessment of Infants and Young Children', in S. Meisels and E. Fenichel (eds), *New Visions for the Developmental Assessment of Infants and Young Children*, Washington, DC: Zero to Three: National Center for Infants, Toddlers and Families.

Guralnick, M. J. (2006) 'Family Influences on Early Development', in K. McCartney and D. Phillips (eds), *Early Childhood Development*. Oxford: Blackwell Publishing, pp. 44–61.

Harrison, L. J. and McLeod, S. (2010) 'Risk and Protective Factors Associated with Speech and Language Impairment in a Nationally Representative Sample of 4 to 5 Year Old Children', *Journal of Speech, Language and Hearing Research* 53: 508–29.

Hertzman, C. (2011) 'Bringing a Population Health Perspective to Early Biodevelopment: An Emerging Approach', in Daniel P. Keating (ed.), *Nature and Nurture in Early Child Development*. New York: Cambridge University Press, pp. 217–44.

Heywood, K. M. and Getchell, N. (2009) *Life Span Motor Development*, 5th edn. Champaign, IL: Human Kinetics, pp. 101–6.

Katz, I. and Pinkerton, J. (2003) *Evaluating Family Support: Thinking Internationally, Thinking Critically*. Chichester: John Wiley & Sons.

Knudsen, E. I. (2004) 'Sensitive Periods in the Development of the Brain and Behavior', *Journal of Cognitive Neuroscience* 16 (8): 1412–25.

Lerner, R. M., Lewin-Bezan, S. and Warren, A. E. A. (2011) 'Concepts and

Theories of Human Development', in M. H. Bornstein and M. E. Lamb (eds), *Cognitive Development: An Advanced Textbook*. New York: Psychology Press, pp. 19–66.

Lindsay, G. and Dockrell, J. (2012) 'The Relationship between Speech, Language and Communication Needs (SLCN) and Behavioural, Emotional and Social Difficulties (BESD)', Department for Education Research Report. https://www.education.gov.uk/publications/standard/publication Detail/Page1/DFE-RR247-BCRP6 (accessed 1 June 2013).

Majnemer, A. and Shevell, M. (1995) 'Diagnostic Yield of the Neurologic Assessment of the Developmentally Delayed Child', *Journal of Pediatrics* 127: 193–9.

Martinez-Torteya, C., Anne Bogat, G., von Eye, A. and Levendosky, A. A. (2009) 'Resilience among Children Exposed to Domestic Violence: The Role of Risk and Protective Factors', *Child Development* 80 (2): 562–77.

Mason, J. (1995) *Cultural Competence Self-Assessment Questionnaire: A Manual for Users*. Portland, OR: Portland State University, Research and Training Center on Family Support and Children's Mental Health. http://www.rtc.pdx.edu/PDF/CCSAQ.pdf (accessed 30 July 2013).

Masten, A. S. and Gewirtz, A. H. (2006) 'Vulnerability and Resilience in Early Child Development', in K. McCartney and D. Phillips (eds), *Early Childhood Development*. Oxford: Blackwell Publishing, p. 30.

Moeschler, J. (2008) 'Genetic Evaluation of Intellectual Disability', *Seminars in Pediatric Neurology* 15: 2–9.

Moeschler, J. and Shevell, M. (2006) 'Committee on Genetics. Clinical Genetic Evaluation of the Child with Mental Retardation or Developmental Delays', *Pediatrics* 117: 2304–16.

Munafò, M. R., Durrant, C., Lewis, G. and Flint, J. (2009) 'Gene x Environment Interactions at the Serotonin Transporter Locus', *Biological Psychiatry* 65: 211–19.

National Scientific Council on the Developing Child (2005) *Excessive Stress Disrupts the Architecture of the Developing Brain: Working Paper #3*. Cambridge, MA: National Scientific Council on the Developing Child, Center on the Developing Child at Harvard University. http://developingchild.harvard.edu/index.php/resources/reports_and_working_papers/working_papers/wp3/ (accessed 1 June 2013).

NSPCC (2007) *'It Doesn't Happen to Disabled Children' – Child Protection and Disabled Children*. Report of the National Working Group on Child Protection and Disability. London: NSPCC.

Palfrey, J. S. and Frazer, C. H. (2000) 'Determining the Etiology of Developmental Delay in Very Young Children: What If We Had a Common Internationally Accepted Protocol?', *Journal of Pediatrics* 136: 569–70.

Paulin-Dubois, D., Brooker, I. and Chow, V. (2009) 'The Developmental Origin of Naïve Psychology in Infancy', *Advances in Child Development and Behaviour* 37: 55–104.

Piek, J. P. (2006) *Infant Motor Development*. Champaign, IL: Human Kinetics.

Robson, P. (1984) 'Prewalking Locomotor Movements and Their Use in Predicting Standing and Walking', *Child Care Health and Development* 10 (5): 317–30

Rogoff, B. (2003) *The Cultural Nature of Human Development*. Oxford: Oxford University Press.

Roulstone, S., Law, J., Rush, R., Clegg, J. and Peters, T. (2011) *Investigating the Role of Language in Children's Early Educational Outcomes*. London: Department for Education, Research Report DFE-RR134, pp. 3, 33–4. https://www.education.gov.uk/publications/eOrderingDownload/DFE-RR134.pdf (accessed 1 June 2013).

Rutter, M. (2006) *Genes and Behaviour: Nature–Nurture Interplay Explained*. Oxford: Blackwell Publishing.

Rutter, M. (2011) 'Biological and Experiential Influences on Psychological Development', in Daniel P. Keating (ed.), *Nature and Nurture in Early Child Development*. New York: Cambridge University Press, pp. 7–44.

Rutter, M. (2013) 'Annual Research Review: Resilience – Clinical Implications', *Journal of Child Psychology and Psychiatry* 54 (4): 474–87.

Sameroff, A. J. (2009) *The Transactional Model of Development: How Children and Contexts Shape Each Other*. Washington, DC: American Psychological Association.

Sameroff, A. J. and Fiese, B. H. (2000) 'Transactional Regulation and Early Intervention', in J. S. Meisels and J. P. Shonkoff (eds), *Handbook of Early Childhood Intervention*, 2nd edn. New York: Cambridge University Press, pp. 119–49.

Sameroff, A. J., Seifer, R. and Baldwin, A. (1993) 'Stability of Intelligence from Preschool to Adolescence: The Influence of Social and Family Risk Factors', *Child Development* 64 (1): 80–97.

Shonkoff, J. P. and Phillips, D. A. (eds) (2000) *From Neurons to Neighborhoods: The Science of Early Childhood Development*, Committee on Integrating the Science of Early Childhood Development. Washington, DC: National Academy Press.

Shonkoff, J. P., Garner, A. S. and The Committee on Psychosocial Aspects of Child and Family Health, Committee on Early Childhood, Adoption, and Dependent Care, and Section on Developmental and Behavioral Paediatrics (2012) 'Technical Report: The Lifelong Effects of Early Childhood Adversity and Toxic Stress', *Pediatrics* 129 (1): e232–46.

Snowling, M. L., Bishop, D. V., Stothard, S. E., Chipchase, B. and Kaplan, C. (2006) 'Psychosocial Outcomes at 15 Years of Children with a

Preschool History of Speech-Language Impairment', *Journal of Child Psychology and Psychiatry* 47 (8): 759–65.

Sroufe, L. A. (2005) 'Attachment and Development: A Prospective, Longitudinal Study from Birth to Adulthood', *Attachment & Human Development* 7 (4): 349–67.

Super, C. M. and Harkness, S. (1997) 'The Cultural Structuring of Child Development', in J. W. Berry, P. S. Dasen and T. S. Saraswathi (eds), *Handbook of Cross-Cultural Psychology, Vol. 2: Basic Processes and Human Development*, 2nd edn. Needham Heights, MA: Allyn & Bacon, pp. 1–40.

Tervo, R. C. (2005) 'Parent's Reports Predict their Child's Developmental Problems', *Clinical Pediatrics* 44: 601–11.

Tervo, R. C. (2006) 'Identifying Patterns of Developmental Delays Can Help Diagnose Neurodevelopmental Disorders', *Clinical Pediatrics* 45: 509–17.

Thelen, E. and Smith, L. (2006) 'Dynamic System Theories', in W. Damon (series ed.) and R. M. Lerner (vol. ed.), *Handbook of Child Psychology: Vol. 1. Theoretical Models of Human Development*, 5th edn. New York: Wiley, pp. 563–633.

Thompson, R. A., Virmani, V. A., Waters, S. F., Abigail Raikes, H. and Meyer, S. (2013) 'The Development of Emotion Self-Regulation: The Whole and the Sum of Parts, in K. C. Barret, N. A. Fox, G. Morgan, D. Fidler and L. Daunhauer (eds), *Handbook of Self-regulatory Processes in Development: New Directions and International Perspectives*. Hove: Psychology Press, pp. 5–26.

Toriello, H. (2008) 'Role of the Dysmorphologic Evaluation in the Child with Developmental Delay', *Pediatric Clinics of North America* 55: 1085–98.

Webster-Stratton, C. and Taylor, T. (2001) 'Nipping Risk Factors in the Bud: Preventing Substance Abuse, Delinquency and Violence in Adolescence through Interventions Targeted at Young Children (0–8 Years)', *Prevention Science* 2 (3): 165–92.

Wellman, H. M. (2004) 'Understanding the Psychological World: Developing a Theory of Mind', in U. Goswami (ed.), *Blackwell Handbook of Childhood Cognitive Development*. Oxford: Blackwell Publishing, pp. 167–87.

Youth Justice Board for England and Wales (2005) 'Risk and Protective Factors'. http://www.yjb.gov.uk/publications/resources/downloads/rpf%20report.pdf (accessed 28 July 2103).

Zeigler, E. and Hodapp, R. M. (1986) *Understanding Mental Retardation*. New York: Cambridge University Press.

Zenah, C. H., Berlin, L. J. and Boris, N. W. (2011) 'Practitioner Review: Clinical Applications of Attachment Theory and Research for Infants and Young Children', *Journal of Child Psychology and Psychiatry* 52 (8): 819–33.

# Pictures to support examination of verbal and non-verbal skills

1. Knowledge of body parts

2. Common objects

   ■ understanding/use of common nouns (*cup, ball, spoon, sock*)

   ■ understanding/use of objects by function (which one do we *drink from/eat with/wear/play with?*)

3. Common actions

   ■ understanding/use of common verbs (*drink, jump, sleep, eat*)

4. Common descriptive concepts

   ■ understanding/use of common adjectives (*big/little, happy/sad, full/empty*)

5. Common spatial concepts

   ■ understanding/use of prepositions (*in, under, behind, on*)

6. Simple narrative – 'naughty dog!'

   ■ ability to connect events to form a narrative

   ■ understanding of common emotions (happy, angry)

   ■ focus for conversation – what will happen next?, do you have any pets? . . .

7. Number and quantity

   ■ counting

   ■ concepts of *more/less*

8. Colour template available for printing

   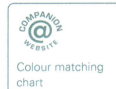

   Colour matching chart

   ■ colour matching (placing coloured shapes/cubes on the matching template)

   ■ understanding/use of colour names

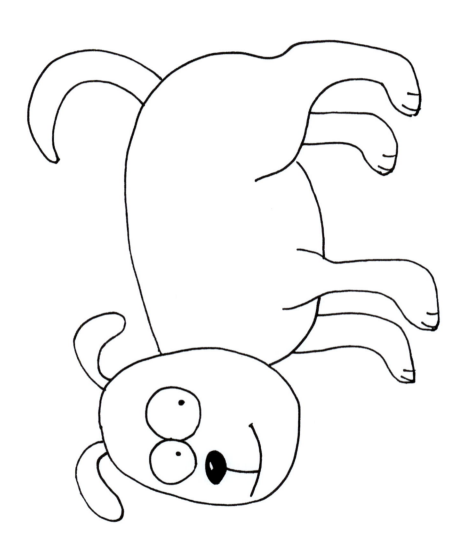

1.

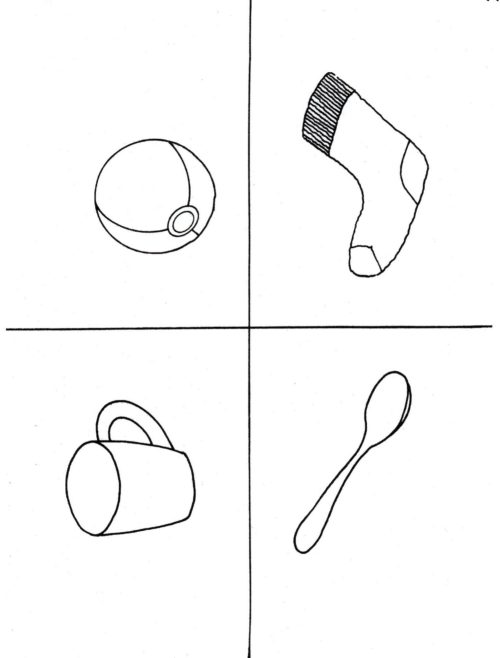

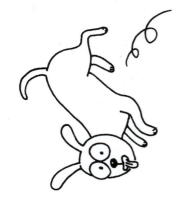
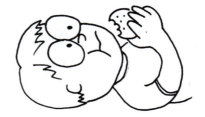
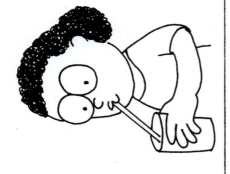
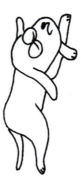

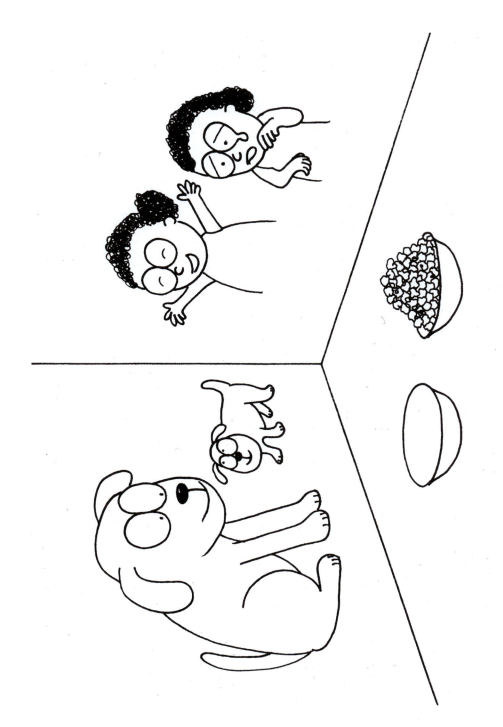

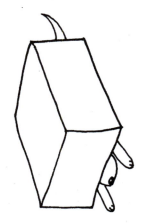
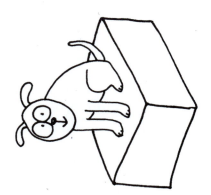
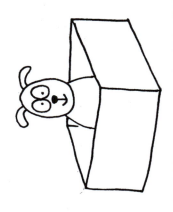
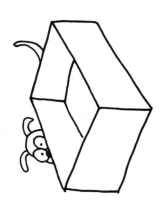

2

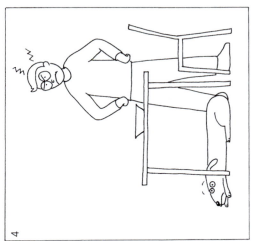

4

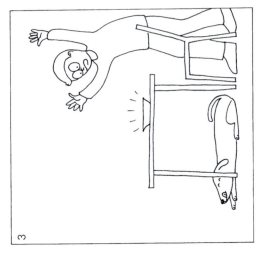

1

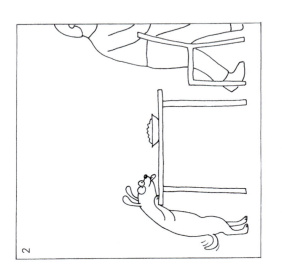

3

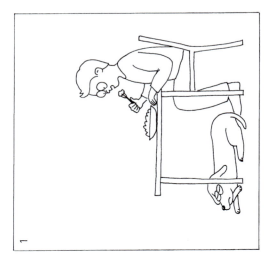

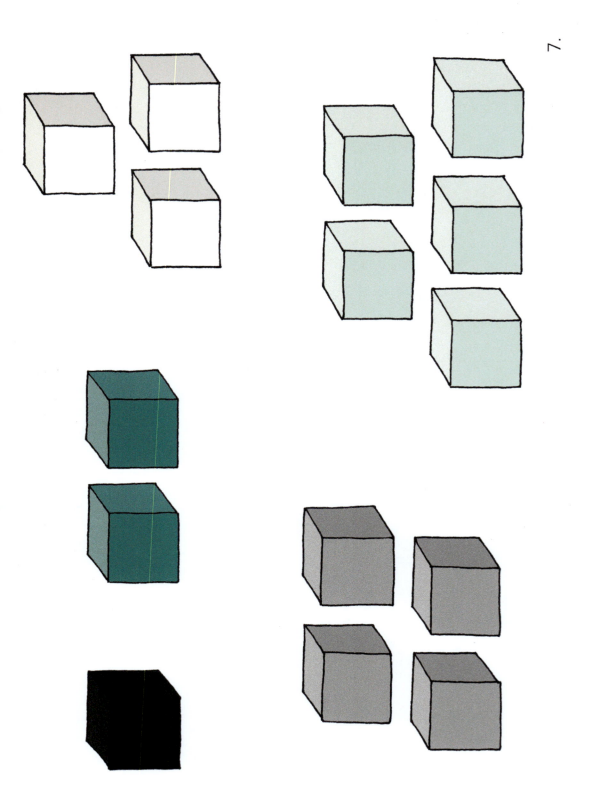